COMMANDO CARDIO

PERFORMANCE-BASED ENERGY OUTPUT
THAT CREATES A METABOLIC DEMAND

JON BRUNEY

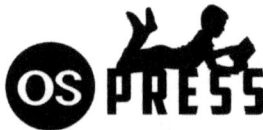

Published by OS Press - Fuquay-Varina, NC

ISBN: 978-1-64184-621-9 (Paperback)
ISBN: 978-1-64184-622-6 (Ebook)

Thank you to Vikki Harris for editing
Thank you to JETLAUNCH.net for book design

Table of Contents

Disclaimer!

You must get your physician's approval before beginning this exercise program. These recommendations are not medical guidelines but are for educational purposes only. You must consult your physician prior to starting this program or if you have any medical condition or injury that is contraindicated to performing physical activity. This program is designed for healthy individuals eighteen years and older only.

See your physician before starting any exercise or nutrition program. If you are taking any medications, you must talk to your physician before starting any exercise program, including Commando Cardio. If you experience any lightheadedness, dizziness, or shortness of breath while exercising, stop the movement and consult a physician.

It is strongly recommended that you have a complete physical examination if you live a sedentary lifestyle, have high cholesterol, high blood pressure, diabetes, are overweight, or if you are over thirty years old. Please discuss all nutritional changes with your physician or a registered dietician. If your physician recommends that you not use Commando Cardio, please follow your doctor's orders.

All forms of exercise pose some inherent risks. The authors, editors, and publishers advise readers to take full responsibility for their safety and know their limits. When using the exercises in this program, do not take risks beyond your level of experience, aptitude, training, and fitness. The exercises and dietary programs in this book are not intended as a substitute for any exercise routine, treatment, or dietary regimen prescribed by your physician.

Read This First

You do not have to own a Neuro-Burner (which is a specialized piece of equipment designed for Commando Cardio protocols) to start this program or apply its principles. You can use beach towels, a piece of canvas, moving blankets, or tarps. Never let the lack of equipment get in the way of your training! Get creative and get training.

Why Commando Cardio?

t's the question new trainees most frequently ask me . . . "What about cardio, bro?" If their definition of cardio is like most people, spending a half an hour on an elliptical machine or treadmill, I tell them, "You don't need it!" They are usually shocked at my answer. They don't need traditional cardio and neither do you!

If you want:

- scarred heart tissue

- a faster aging body due to free radical damage

- a larger appetite

- less muscle

- more fat

- to waste time

Then by all means, make sure you do all the traditional steady-state cardio you can.

What we all need is proper physical conditioning. I remember in my early days going to Gold's Gym and watching guys spend hours on the stair climber (the stair climber was all the rage in the early 90's) after their weightlifting sessions trying to get "ripped." They were ripping alright; they were actually ripping off their hard-earned muscle. Yes, I have seen bodybuilders and powerlifters who were poorly conditioned. But, traditional, steady-state cardio is not the best option for increased conditioning.

Steady-state cardio is not the best option for increased conditioning.

When I served as a trainer on a weight-loss/transformation local cable television show, I had the privilege of helping some great people make some serious changes to their body composition. I understood their frustration as they signed up for the show. Many of them had been performing hours of steady-state cardio for quite some time. The problem was that in spite of all that cardio, they were actually getting fatter. Their workouts had sapped their muscle and strength. Fortunately, I was able to show them a better way.

Do athletes need steady-state cardio? Unless they are endurance based, my answer would still be no. Commando Cardio will lay a blueprint for athletes to increase their work capacity, tolerate lactate, and increase athleticism.

I believe it's possible to even increase endurance without steady-state cardio. When I wanted to run a 5k race for my birthday, I didn't train for it by jogging miles a day. Besides my weight training, I did Commando Cardio. The result: I had no problem running the race.

It's time to break free from the belief you need hours of cardio a week to be healthy. Have you ever seen an elephant in a circus? Elephants have a rope or chain tied around one their legs and attached to a small stake in the ground. You may wonder why the elephant never rips the stake out of the ground and roams off. After all, with the elephant's power, it could easily break free. The reason is the elephant doesn't know it can break free. When the elephant is still a baby, trainers chain it every night to a tree. The baby elephant will try with all its power to break the chain. The baby elephant will try over and over to break free without success. After many attempts the elephant gives up, believing that it is impossible to ever be free. Once the elephant is conditioned to believe it can't break free, it will never try again for the rest of its life. So many people are conditioned to believe that if they don't do steady-state cardio they'll die of heart disease or get fat. It's time to rip that stake out of the ground.

I will show you a better way.

I have trained NFL players and Olympic athletes. I also have trained people who just want to get in better shape. I apply the principles of Commando Cardio with all of them.

Why? Because it works! This is not a textbook on aerobics. This is a battle-tested, in-the-trenches methodology that has been successful for all who have embraced it. And not only does it work, but it takes minimal equipment and can be done **This is not a textbook on aerobics.** virtually anywhere. If you are ready for an all-out assault on your conditioning… Get ready for Commando Cardio!

Commando Cardio – Producing Superior Results!

Commando Cardio: Performance-Based Energy Output That Creates a Metabolic Demand. This type of training raises your *metabolic rate* through high lactate and increased oxygen intake. Following a Commando Cardio session, the body has to repay its oxygen debt. This creates an effect called EPOC: excess post-exercise oxygen consumption. The EPOC effect causes the body to continue to burn calories long after the training session is finished.

A Surge Set is an intense bout of exercise done for a short period of time.

This is accomplished through the implementation of *Surge Sets*. A Surge Set is an intense bout of exercise done for a short period of time. The sets are all-out, powerful bursts. Just like a wave in the ocean, a Surge Set starts powerfully and affects everything in its path. Just as a wave gets smaller as it comes in to shore, a Surge Set ends as soon as the intensity drops.

These explosive bursts of energy with strategically timed rest periods are what makes Commando Cardio so effective.

The all-out intensity of Surge Sets produces lactic acid in the bloodstream. This causes the body to go through a process of producing growth hormone to help the body recover and adapt. This natural production of growth hormone is one of the reasons why Commando Cardio is so powerful. Here are just some of the benefits you may receive as a result of increased growth hormone levels.

Decreased body fat

Growth hormone triggers fat cells to be used for energy. Most people rely on glucose for energy. By raising growth hormone through the exercise protocols in Commando Cardio your body will begin to use fat as its fuel of choice. This means you will become a fat burning machine, even while sleeping. Growth hormone production combined with the afterburn metabolic effect of Surge Sets will cause rapid body re-composition.

Surge Sets will cause rapid body re-composition.

Increased lean muscle mass

Growth hormone aids in protein synthesis. This is the process of repairing and building muscle tissue. Simply put, growth hormone assists in speeding up this muscle recovery process. During this recovery phase the body increases lean mass. Since muscle burns calories to maintain itself, this results in even more around the clock fat burning.

Anti-aging

To understand the aging process, we need to look at telomeres and healthy cells. The human body's chromosomes have telomeres attached to their ends. The role of the telomere is to protect the chromosome and to keep other chromosomes from connecting to them. When the chromosome replicates through cell division, part of the telomere is lost or shortened.

Eventually the process of telomere shortening decreases the length of the cell so that it no longer has the ability to replicate. When the cells can no longer replicate, the cells age and eventually die. Aging cells = aging body. Scientists are now looking at telomere length as an indicator of where your body is in the aging process. What if there was a way to slow the process of telomere shortening and maintain cellular health? New cutting edge research is showing that healthy growth hormone levels produced through high intensity exercise can help preserve telomere length. Surge sets can help slow the aging process and ward off disease. Commando Cardio may be your ticket to the fountain of youth.

Aging cells = aging body.

Increased sex drive and performance

Testosterone is the hormone that increases sexual interest. Many couples are not in the mood or too distracted for intimate relations. One of the key reasons this may be occurring is hormonal. Low levels of testosterone are shown can cause low libido, irritability, anxiety, and decrease in motivation. Growth hormone can help alleviate the symptoms of low testosterone. Numerous studies show that increasing growth hormone levels will also increase testosterone levels. This occurs because growth hormone works as an overall regulating hormone in the body.

Also, the added benefits of decreased body fat, body re-composition, increased conditioning levels, and positive mental outlook resulting from Surge Sets may breathe new life into your intimate relationship.

Bone density maintenance

Bone mass begins to decline when the body is in the thirties. We have all heard about individuals breaking a hip or experiencing some catastrophic injury in their senior years due to weakened bones. Who can forget the famous "I've Fallen and I Can't get up!" commercial? Increased growth hormone stimulates I-GF1 and Gla Protein both which can help maintain the density of your bones. The effect is greater amounts of calcium and osteocalcin in the bones which reduces the risk of fracture. Healthy bones are essential to your fitness and performance goals.

Healthy bones are essential to your fitness and performance goals.

Relief from the symptoms of anxiety and depression

Depression affects nearly everyone at some point in their lifetime. The reasons for depression and anxiety are many. Loss of job, relationship issues, stress, finances, and a whole host of other problems tend to block out hope. Growth hormone is nature's anti-depressant. By raising the level of the neurotransmitter B-endorphin, individuals have increased feelings of well-being and self-confidence. The intense exercise protocols in Commando Cardio may be a missing link in improving mental health.

Better skin and a more youthful appearance

Aging causes a loss of skin elasticity and thickness, leading to wrinkles and a loss of skin tone. Growth hormone increases the collagen and elastin in the epidermis. This restores strength, texture, and thickness resulting in a younger appearance.

Increased energy levels

Many people are looking for something to help them have enough energy to get through the day. Look at all the energy shot products advertised everywhere. Growth hormone has been linked to higher energy levels. Higher energy allows for opportunities to live a fuller life. Less fatigue leads to more motivation to accomplish goals. Get a natural shot of energy by regularly engaging in Surge Sets.

Because of all the benefits that growth hormone has to offer, HGH injections and therapy have become very popular. You will not need to engage in dangerous injections or get a prescription. The Commando Cardio program will help you stimulate growth hormone naturally, so you get all the benefits and none of the negative side effects.

> **Higher energy allows for opportunities to live a fuller life.**

Short sessions

Short sessions are very important because they allow you to save your hard-earned muscle. Long cardio sessions can eat up your muscle tissue through the release of too much cortisol. Cortisol also causes inflammation, and can even decrease the effectiveness of the thyroid. Commando Cardio saves your muscles and your time. With more time, you can focus on practicing your skill, sport, or hobby. Most elite athletes must spend time developing a specific skill set. Commando Cardio doesn't drain your time, so you have more time to focus on what is most important to your training and athletic goals.

> **Commando Cardio saves your muscles and your time.**

Performance-based

That's right, these training sessions will actually increase your performance. The exercises in Commando Cardio have great carryover to most sports. Commando Cardio also increases performance by creating a neural boost. Explosive exercises are shown to have the ability to wake up the nervous system. This causes more muscle fibers to fire allowing you to jump higher, lift heavier, or run faster. Here are just some of the many other performance enhancing benefits from Commando Cardio:

- Increased lactate threshold. You will increase your body's ability to handle high levels of lactate, important for most sports and competitions.

- Increased ability to recover quickly after strenuous practices, games, or meets

- Stronger heart with increased lung capacity. This translates to greater endurance and work capacity.

- Smarter body from teaching the body to perform opposing dynamic movements

- Increased speed and velocity

- More resistance to injuries

Physically and mentally challenging

Traditional cardio is boring! It becomes mindless and mundane. That's why so many people watch TV while on the treadmill or elliptical. The lack of variety in traditional cardio also means that the body adapts and is no longer challenged. No wonder people struggle to stay motivated while performing traditional cardio. Commando Cardio will engage the mind and challenge the body. The variety of progressions will keep your workouts fresh and continually push your conditioning limits.

Traditional cardio is boring!

Helps maintain overall health

The training methods used in Commando Cardio have been shown to prevent diseases and encourage healthy eating patterns. The program prevents diabetes by helping with insulin sensitivity. Surge Set type training also lowers the risk of cardiovascular disease by helping to control hypertension and hardening of the arteries.

Traditional steady state cardio has been shown to create increase appetite for food. This means that the calories burned in that long elliptical session may end up being consumed post workout. Commando Cardio assists in healthy eating by releasing hormones that make you feel full while also suppressing hunger signals.

The benefits of Commando Cardio over steady-state cardio are numerous. But, there is something that sets Commando Cardio apart from the rest of the pack ... it can be done almost anywhere with minimal equipment.

That's where the name Commando Cardio comes from. Commandos are often placed in remote areas, with **Minimalist, portable, intense, and results orientated.** minimal equipment, and high expectations of results. Their missions also involve getting in, getting the job done, and getting out. I am no Commando, but I wanted a conditioning program that had those same ideals: *minimalist, portable, intense, and results orientated.*

Requires minimal equipment

There are many great conditioning weapons in the competitive athlete's arsenal. Two of my favorites are kettlebells and the battling ropes. Kettlebells are an excellent form of conditioning. The problem is that I can't throw a kettlebell in my backpack. **One of the cornerstones of Commando Cardio is sustained speed, better defined as velocity.**

The battling ropes are also an exceptional way to perform cardio work. I am a Level 2 Battling Ropes Coach. John Brookfield, the creator of the system, is my mentor. The problem with the ropes is that they require a large area to work with. A good 25-30 foot minimum distance from the anchor point is required to use the ropes effectively. A 50 ft. 2 inch diameter rope definitely can be a portability issue.

Fortunately, there is a way to get all the cardio benefits of kettlebell and battling ropes training with minimal portable implements.

One of the cornerstones of Commando Cardio is sustained speed, better defined as velocity. I have had the privilege of learning velocity exercise techniques from eminent trainers Ori Hofmekler and John Brookfield. Commando Cardio builds upon these basic ideas by adding progressions, protocols, and performance maximizers. There are many different inexpensive implements that can accommodate the demands of this system.

Some good choices are: heavy beach towels, canvas, moving blankets, yoga mats, and parachute material. I designed a piece of equipment for this program called the Neuro-Burner, but it is not necessary to have one.

Different implements will provide different levels of resistance.

Different implements will provide different levels of resistance. Experiment with different tools until you find out what works best for you.

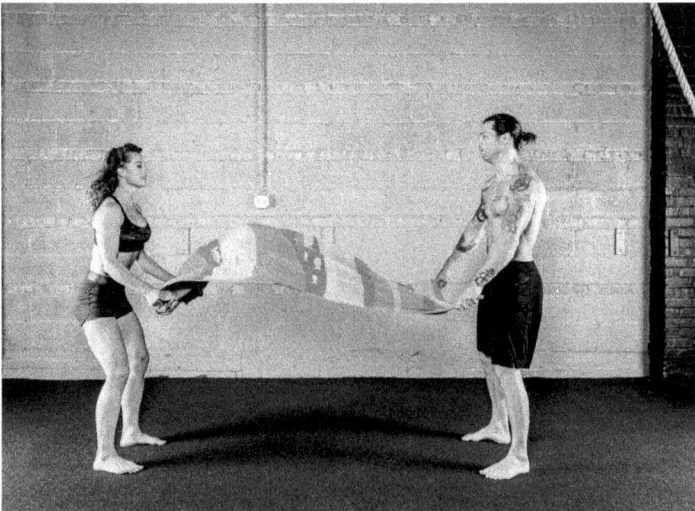

The Power of a Partner

"One is too small a number to achieve greatness."

-John Maxwell

I f you want to get the most out of the Commando Cardio system, you will want to invest some time into a finding a training partner. Performing Commando Cardio with a partner will maximize your results, taking you to an extraordinary level of conditioning. Here are just a few of the benefits of training partnerships:

Competition

We all have at some level, a competitive spirit. The Surge Sets in Commando Cardio create an opportunity to "battle" and compete with a partner. Who will provide the most resistance? Who can keep up the intensity? Who will tap out first? These little battles create great conditioning sessions.

We all have at some level, a competitive spirit.

I know that when I train with my lifting partners, there is always a competition to see who is going to set the pace for the workout. Everyone wants to do one more rep than the others for the evenings bragging rights. The result is that everyone is pushed to a higher level of intensity.

The competitive nature of Commando Cardio will drive you to want to go one more round. As Rocky Balboa said to Tommy Gunn during Rocky V - "Yo, Tommy! I didn't hear no bell . . ."

Motivation

Even the best athletes will occasionally struggle with motivation. When there are times that you don't "feel" like training, there a several ways having a partner can spark your motivational fire. For starters, there is the accountability factor of knowing that someone has set aside their time to train with you. We don't like to let people down. This helps keep your workouts consistent. Lack of consistency is why most programs fail. Your partner will help you to keep showing up, even when your desire is lacking.

Lack of consistency is why most programs fail.

Another way that a partner motivates is through encouragement. When the workout is getting tough, good workout partners encourage one another to continue to push through the pain. Encouraging statements and attitudes will invigorate your energy and drive.

Technique

Having a training partner also keeps you from having sloppy technique. They will make sure your form is good. Continuing to focus on technique, even when the body is tired, ensures that you will get the best gains from your workout.

Use the "Michael Jordan principle" when choosing a training partner

When choosing a workout partner, I suggest finding someone who is more conditioned than you. Why? Because, if your partner is a better athlete than you, they can help you push to their level of conditioning. I like to think of this as the "Michael Jordan Principle."

Michael Jordan will go down in history as one of the greatest basketball players ever. What does that fact have to do with choosing a training partner? Michael had the ability to elevate the performance of everyone on his team. Players became better just by playing with him! One of those players was Scottie Pippen. Pippen became Jordan's go-to teammate on the Chicago Bulls. They pushed themselves to greatness. The result was that they won 6 championships together and Scottie Pippen became a star in his own right. He was even inducted into the basketball Hall of fame.

So, when choosing a training partner, look for someone who:

- Is at a higher level of physical conditioning.

- Has a competitive attitude.

- Will hold you accountable.

- Is positive.

- Is consistent in their training.

I have always tried to learn from others whose skills and abilities were better than mine. Whether it was in athletics, writing, speaking, business, coaching, or leadership, I always have tried to partner with those who were at a higher level. I owe much of my success to the many individuals who invested in my growth.

I have always tried to learn from others whose skills and abilities were better than mine.

Find a partner and watch your conditioning soar!

Rare Air – Reaping the Benefits of Resisted Breathing and the Carbon Dioxide Conditioning Paradox

Warning- the following techniques are to be performed at your own risk!

One of the methods that athletes have used to increase conditioning and sports performance is altitude training. In high altitudes the air contains less oxygen. As the athletes become more accustomed to the lower oxygen levels, bodily changes occur. One is increased concentration of red blood cells due the production of the erythropoietin (EPO) hormone. EPO triggers red blood cell production in the body. Red blood cells ferry oxygen to the muscles. This transfer of oxygen to the muscles provides better endurance and performance.

Several other beneficial changes also occurred including a lowered heart rate while performing physical exertion. Another adaption was an increased ability to buffer lactic acid. Overall, the body becomes much more efficient in performing exercise.

We can partially simulate altitude training with the Commando Cardio program by using a breathing resistance device during Surge Sets. These devices provide resistance against inspiration. In other words, they work by limiting the amount of air that can be inhaled. This helps strengthen and develop the lungs and diaphragm. However, these devices do not lower the actual oxygen content of the air as in higher elevations.

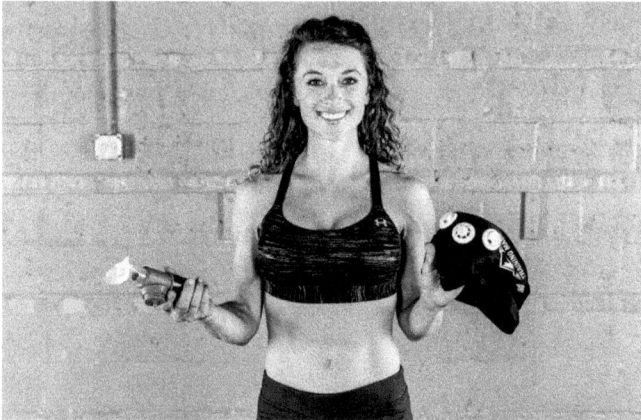

The solution- carbon dioxide enrichment. Carbon dioxide enrichment can be added to the program to oxygenate the body and take the conditioning effect even further. It is a paradox…strategically increasing carbon dioxide to increase oxygen levels. According to Dr. Artour Rakhimov, "CO2 is a powerful dilator of blood vessels and is essential for oxygen release in tissues (The Bohr law)." Listen to what Ray Peat, Ph.D. says, "Breathing pure oxygen lowers the oxygen content of tissues; breathing rarefied air, or air with carbon dioxide, oxygenates and energizes the tissues; if this seems upside down, it's because medical physiology has been taught upside down."

The solution- carbon dioxide enrichment.

Here's why it works:

First, carbon dioxide works with red blood cells, increasing the hemoglobin's sensitivity to oxygen. This results in the ability to transport oxygen more efficiently.

Second, when the carbon dioxide content of the blood is elevated, the arteries and blood vessels expand to allow for more blood and oxygen flow.

Third, carbon dioxide helps to regulate PH in the blood. Proper PH levels are critical to keeping the body oxygenated.

If you want to start a carbon dioxide enrichment protocol, first clear it with your doctor. If you have cerebrovascular problems, heart disease, or have suffered a stroke, this technique isn't for you.

Once you are cleared, you will need a small paper bag. Using your hands, attach the bag around your nose and mouth. Begin inhaling and exhaling into the bag. You will start to take in carbon dioxide because you are rebreathing your exhaled air. Continue inhaling and exhaling for thirty seconds. Immediately stop if you get dizzy or experience any negative side effects. This breathing protocol should be done several times throughout the day. It is a good idea to have someone watching you when performing this technique. Carbon dioxide enrichment should be done at a *separate time* from your Commando Cardio sessions.

These techniques work! I have had great success with these protocols. Several years ago, I had a series of strength shows in Cheyenne, Wyoming. Prior to the trip, I was warned about the low oxygen content of the location where I would be performing. Because I regularly use these techniques, I had no problems. During that trip I had some of the best performances of my career.

Incorporate resisted breathing and carbon dioxide enrichment into your program and reap the benefits of elite conditioning levels.

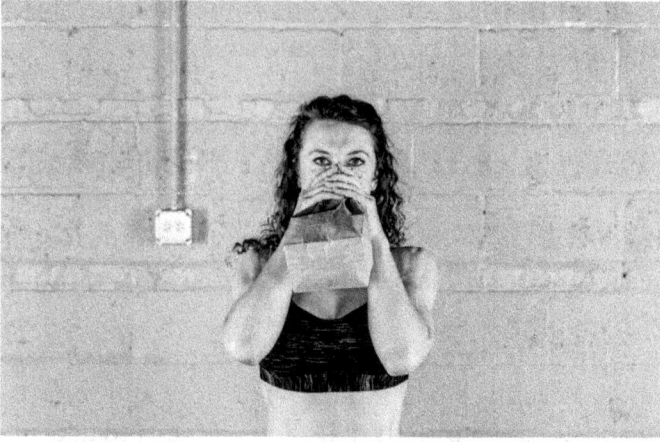

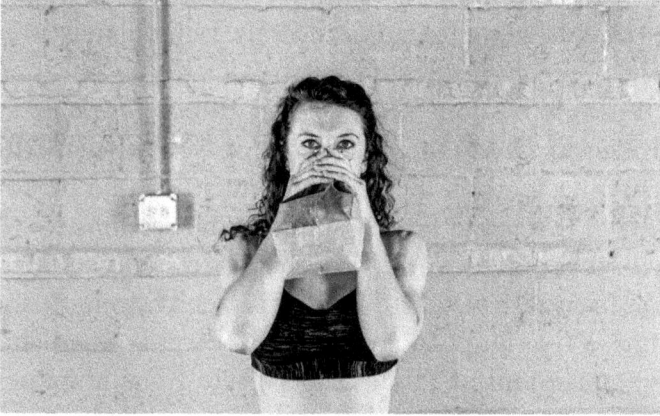

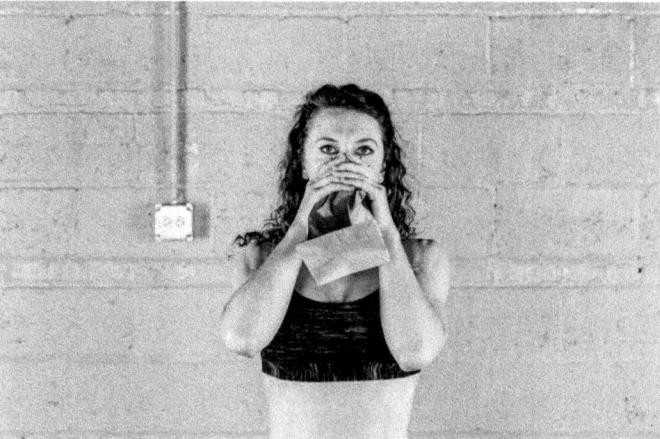

Gaining a Nutritional Edge

Good nutrition can enhance any physical fitness program. There are ways to supplement your healthy diet that can complement your conditioning sessions. Be advised that there is no magic pill that will transform your physique and abilities. Too many people are looking for a fitness shortcut in a bottle. There is no substitute for hard work and clean eating. However, if you are looking for supplements that will work synergistically with your training, here are some to consider:

> **There is no substitute for hard work and clean eating.**

Vitamin D3 and K2

The "Sunshine Vitamin" D3 can be produced by the body through exposure to the sun. However, many individuals do not spend enough time in the sun to produce optimal amounts of vitamin D, due to work environments, school, and geography.

Vitamin D3 is essential to allowing the body repair and recover. D3 supplementation has been shown to boost a myriad of the body's biological mechanisms including; assisting DNA repair, boosting the immune system, and cardiovascular health.

Vitamin D3 acts as a steroid hormone in the body and can increase testosterone levels. Optimal hormone levels are one of the keys to getting the most out of your training program. Proper D3 levels help to ensure that your body is performing at its best.

If you choose to use supplemental D3, make sure to pair it with vitamin K2. Vitamin D3 increases the body's ability to absorb more calcium. K2 allows calcium to be deposited in your skeletal system instead of the other areas of the body where it could be detrimental to your health.

Before beginning a D3 and K2 supplement protocol, get you levels checked by a doctor. It is estimated that a majority of the population is vitamin D3 deficient.

Recommendation if you are deficient:

D3: 5,000 to 8,000 IU per day. I like to divide the doses equally starting in the morning. I take the second dose later in the evening or post workout. If you are taking too much D3, you will develop a metallic aftertaste in your mouth. If this side-effect occurs, stop the supplemental protocol immediately.

K2: 100-150 MCG

L-carnitine tartrate

Carnitine is an excellent addition to your Commando Cardio program. One of the biggest benefits is that it helps the body to burn fat. L-carnitine has also been shown to improve athletic performance by reducing physical and mental fatigue. L-carnitine tartrate acts as a transporter of fat to be used for energy. This means that you will burn more fat, have more energy, and improve body composition. This is definitely a nutrient you want in your dietary arsenal.

Recommendation:

L-Carnitine Tartrate: 1500-2000 mg daily

L-taurine

Supplementing with taurine can assist in dilating the vascular system. Taurine causes the body to excrete nitric oxide. Nitric oxide increases blood flow and delivery of oxygen to the muscles. Taurine also protects the body against free radical damage.

I have also experienced greater mental focus during workouts while ingesting L-taurine. It is a great supplement that will charge up your conditioning workouts.

Recommendation:

L-taurine: 1000 mg pre-workout

L-citrulline

L-citrulline is another powerful tool in vasodilation. Supplemental L-citrulline enters the kidneys and then converts to the amino acid L-arginine. The body uses L-arginine to produce nitric oxide. The boost of nitric oxide as already stated, increases blood and oxygen flow to the muscles. Citrulline also reduces fatigue by helping the body to clear out ammonia during workouts.

L-citrulline has become a staple in my nutrition regimen. After years of searching out the best vasodilation supplements, I have personally found L-citrulline to be the most effective.

Recommendation:

L-citrulline: 3000-6000 mg pre-workout

Fish oil

I saved the best individual supplement for last. There are so many benefits to ingesting fish oil that entire books have been written about it. I want to highlight a few of the benefits that relate to conditioning. Fish oil has been shown to increase the body's ability to burn fat when combined with exercise. Another key benefit is the anti-inflammatory effect that occurs when fish oil is taken at the proper doses. The final benefit that applies to the Commando Cardio program is muscle sparing. Multiple studies have shown that fish oil helps to preserve lean muscle mass. Protecting your muscle while on a conditioning program is essential to continued progress.

Recommendation:

Fish oil: 1400 mg daily

The Commando Cardio Daily Detox and Performance Booster Shake:

Every morning I start my day with a nutrient dense shake. To create this powerhouse drink, you will need a high powered blender. Add water to your desired consistency. The thickness of the shake is up to your personal preference.
Ingredients:

- 1 scoop of powdered greens mix
- 20 grams of whey protein
- Beet root extract powder
- Probiotic powder

This shake will energize you for the upcoming day. Try it and make the most out of your morning nutrition.

The Velocity Swipe – The Foundational Movement in Commando Cardio

"The more I train, the more I realize I have more speed in me."

-Leroy Burrell

The velocity swipe is the antithesis of slow and steady aerobic training. This foundational exercise in the Commando Cardio will not only develop world class conditioning, but explosive speed also. The ability to explode with powerful surges of energy over and over will give you an edge over your competition.

Commando Cardio will help you rediscover the lost skill of velocity conditioning. I say rediscover, because you

Commando Cardio will help you rediscover the lost skill of velocity conditioning.

may have performed a version of the velocity swipe way back in elementary school gym class. Other than dodge ball and floor hockey, one of my favorite times in gym class was parachute day.

The teacher would bring out a giant parachute with sets of handles that encircled it. The whole class would grab the handles as the teacher would place balls on the parachute and we would play a game called "Popcorn." The goal was for the class to move the parachute rapidly up and down hard enough that the balls would be bounced off. The game quickly had all of us gasping for breath. What worked then, still works now. Moving explosively up and down against resistance is the foundation that all the Commando Cardio progressions are built upon.

To help you understand why this type of movement is a superior form of conditioning, let's try a simple exercise. Starting with your hands at your sides, explosively propel your arms upward. When they reach the top, let them fall back to your side. Now, you will notice that not a lot of energy was expended and the movement was pretty easy. This time we will try something different. Assume the same starting position as the previous exercise, and explosively drive your hands upward. Now, just as your hands reach eye level, explosively reverse the movement downward. Before your hands reach the starting point reverse them again. Repeat this motion for 15 seconds. You will notice that forcefully changing direction of an explosive movement requires a large amount of energy, engages the whole body, and elevates the heart rate. Imagine how much more these effects are intensified when resistance is added to the movement.

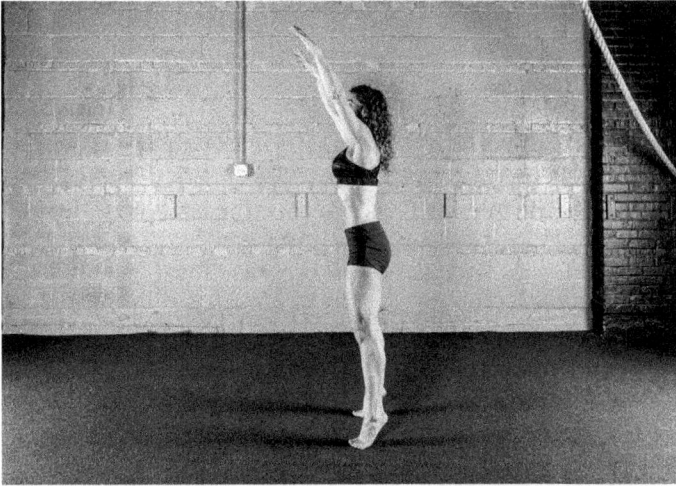

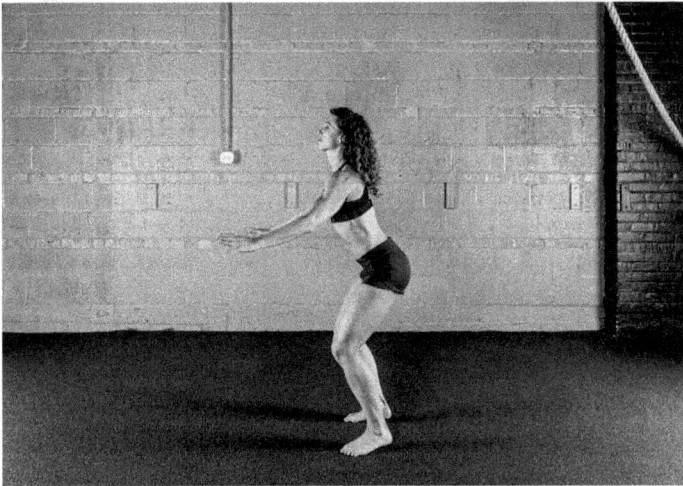

A top fuel dragster race car can travel at speeds in excess of 330 MPH. The 7,000 horsepower engine sends the car screaming down the track. Imagine if it were possible, to take that car at its peak speed forward and quickly send it in reverse. That will give you a mental picture of the power that your body produces when performing the velocity swipe. You are performing an explosive all-out effort in one direction and reversing that movement back quickly with force repeatedly.

Another reason the velocity swipe is foundational to the Commando Cardio program is that it engages the whole body. Even though the upper body is the primary mover in this exercise, the lower body is involved in stabilization. In fact, if the exercise is performed properly, the legs receive a great workout through isometric tension. A freight train traveling at 55 mph takes over a mile of track to stop once the emergency brake is pulled. Now, as the train slows down every car is affected, not just the engine. Think of your body as a train, linked together by the anterior, lateral, and posterior chains. Intense exercise affects all the chains. Unlike the freight train, the velocity swipe doesn't allow for a long distance to slow down and stop. This exercise rapidly changes directions and all the chains in the body must work together to keep the train from derailing. Commando Cardio challenges the stability muscles in the chains, which increases athletic performance.

Intense exercise affects all the chains.

An added benefit from the basic velocity swipe is shoulder health. Shoulder injuries run rampant in the fitness community. A shoulder injury can keep you sidelined from competing in your chosen sport. The rapid whip-like motion of the velocity swipe injury proofs your shoulders in several ways. First of all, the movement restores the "snap" back into the tendons and muscles of the shoulder girdle. Modern training has a plethora of pushing and pulling movements, but very few snapping or whip-like movements. Because this type of training is often ignored, many trainees get injured when they throw, punch, or perform some other power oriented shoulder movement. How many times have you heard of someone "tweaking" their shoulder? The result is lost range of motion, lost time on the field, and lost athletic ability. The velocity swipe will download the "snap" into your body's software, so you can punch harder, throw faster, and always be ready to perform explosively.

The second way is increased circulation to the entire shoulder girdle. The intense energy output of the velocity swipe movement causes the body to shuttle blood and nutrients to the shoulders to help them recover. This extra circulation ensures that the shoulders are receiving the proper amount of nutrients to keep them performing at their best.

The velocity swipe also makes the body smarter because it requires you to do opposing exercises at the same time. Remember when you were a kid the big challenge was to rub your stomach in a circle while patting your head at the same time? The same concept is true here. The beginner progressions of the velocity swipe require the upper body to move dynamically while the lower body is performing an isometric contraction.

Advanced progressions call for the upper body and lower body to perform opposing dynamic movements. By the time you reach that level, you will notice that your body is becoming more efficient and athletic.

Proper technique + Hard work = Great results

You must have proper technique to reap the benefits of the velocity swipe exercise. You can't get lazy with your form. Let's look at the technical aspects of the movement.

To start, the lower body must be tensing in an isometric fashion. Begin by placing your feet shoulder width apart and digging your toes into the ground. Imagine you are at a beach and your feet are digging into the sand. If you are doing this correctly, you should feel tension in your calves and shins.

You can't get lazy with your form.

Now, with the knees slightly bent, move up to the quadriceps and hamstrings. Engage them by flexing hard. Continue to create lower body tension by squeezing your gluteal muscles hard. Tensing the glutes will help to protect the lower back by preventing excessive leaning. By now the whole lower body should be contracting isometrically. The idea is to build a strong base that is actively engaged. Do not hold your breath during the contraction!

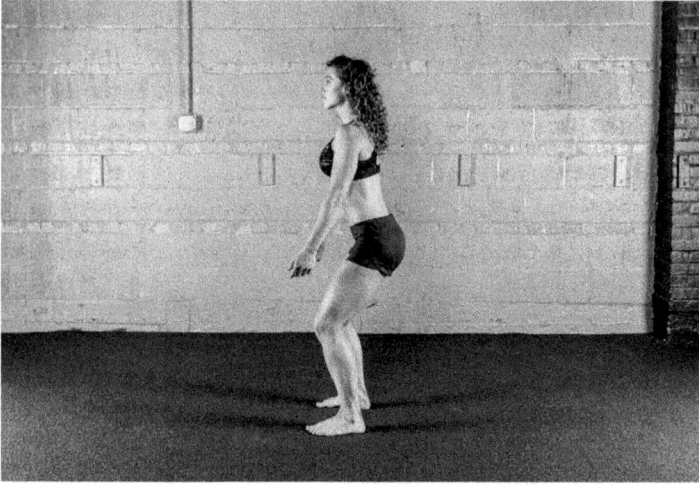

Remember, we are going to be doing conditioning work! Practice holding this lower body isometric contraction until you have mastered the technique.

As we move to the upper body dynamic portion of this exercise, there are several performance points to master. The first is pulling the shoulders back by engaging the scapula. Many trainees attempt to perform the velocity swipe with rounded shoulders. This greatly diminishes the effectiveness of the exercise. Rounding of the shoulders during the velocity swipe can lead to poor posture, shoulder injury, and diminished power output. The best way to get your shoulders into the proper position is by pulling the scapula together. Many athletes struggle with this due to poor lumbar flexibility. Fortunately, there is an effective exercise that will help you learn how to activate and engage the scapula for increased shoulder performance.

The exercise is the "scap-up." Begin by getting into the lockout position of a push-up. Now, keeping the elbows locked lower your upper body toward the floor. You should feel your shoulder blades pushing together. From the bottom position slowly rise upward while keeping the elbows locked. Continue to move upward until the back is rounded. If you are doing the movement correctly, you will feel a great stretch at lower and upper positions of the exercise. The scap-up is an excellent way to warm-up the body for Commando Cardio protocols. If you continue to perform this exercise regularly, you will be rewarded with flexibility and shoulder health that will enhance your everyday life.

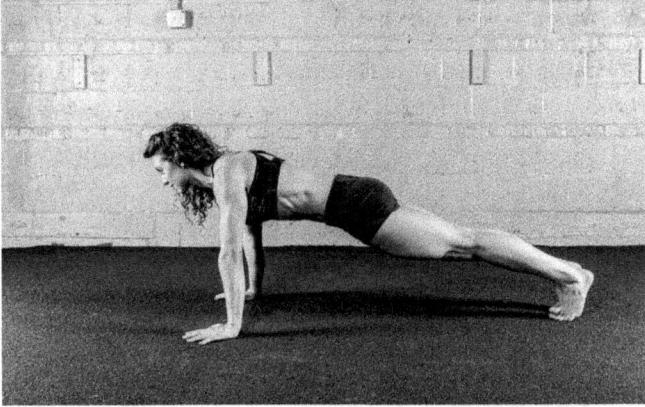

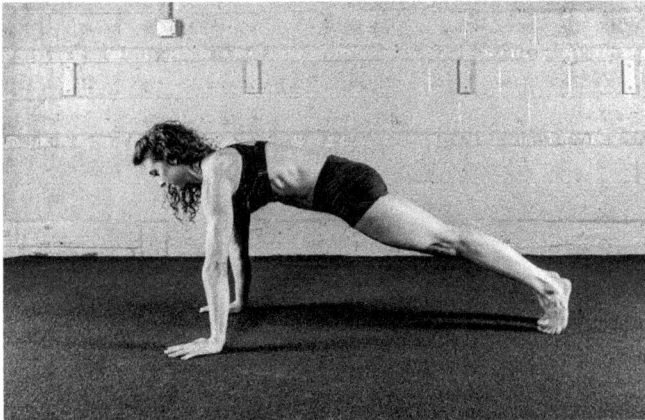

Once you have learned how to isometrically contract the lower body and how to position the upper body, you are ready to perform the movement.

Commando Cardio drills are best performed with a partner. But, what if you don't have a partner? The solution is to attach your implement to a doorway or power rack. There are many different ways to do this using daisy chains or carabiners.

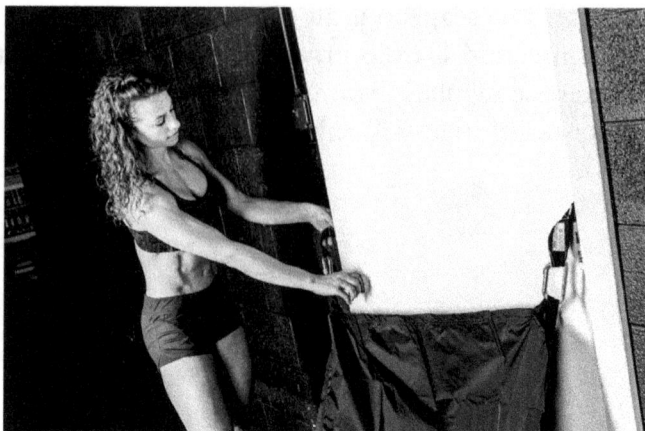

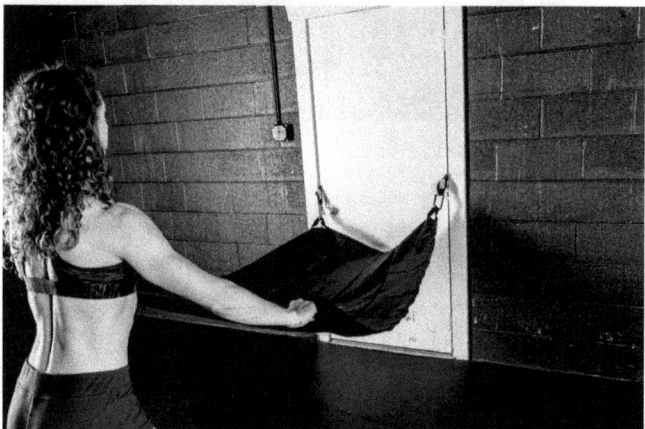

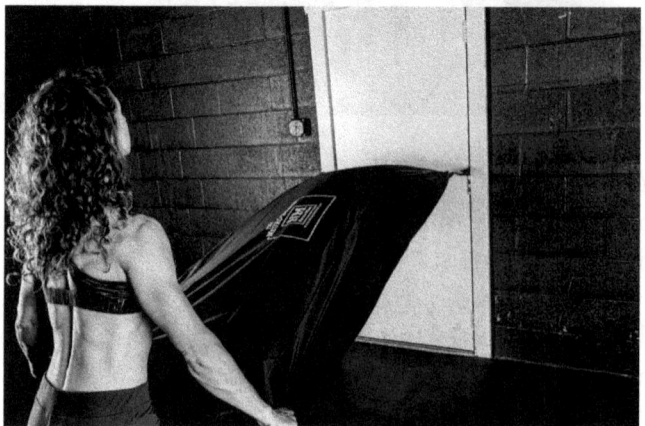

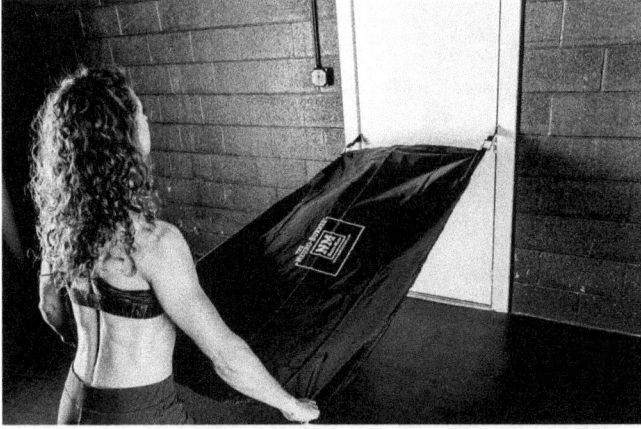

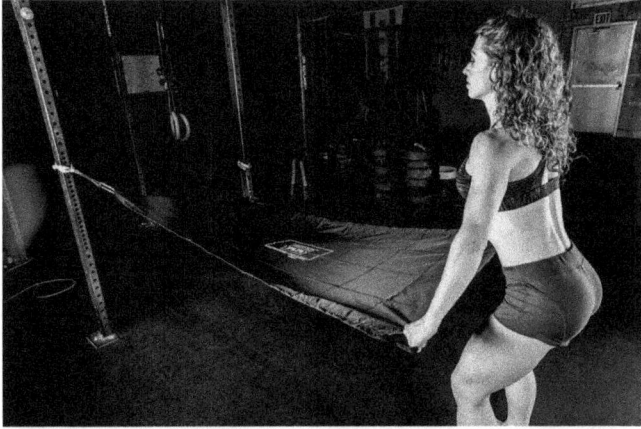

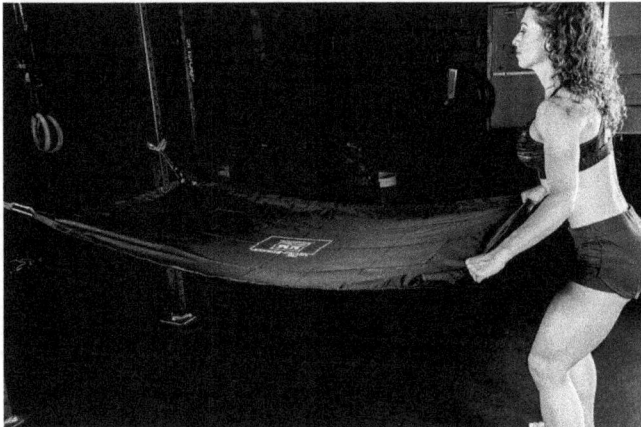

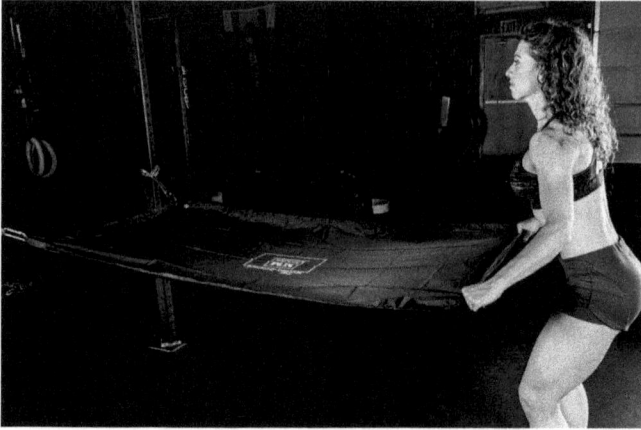

When you are prepared, grasp the handles of your Commando Cardio Implement (referred to from now on as CCI) with your palms facing down and pull them outward until you feel tension. Now, assume the proper distance from your partner or anchor point. Begin to tighten the lower body and pull the shoulders down and back. Rapidly thrust the CCI upward and as soon as it reaches the eye level snap it back down forcefully. Do not let your hands drift inward. Repeat the movement creating as much speed as possible. Continue for 30 seconds.

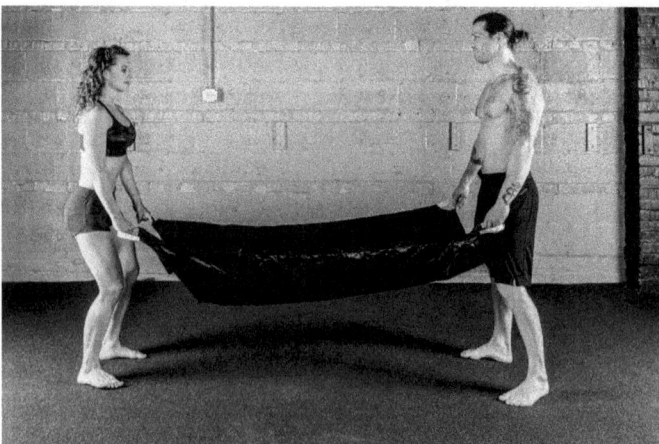

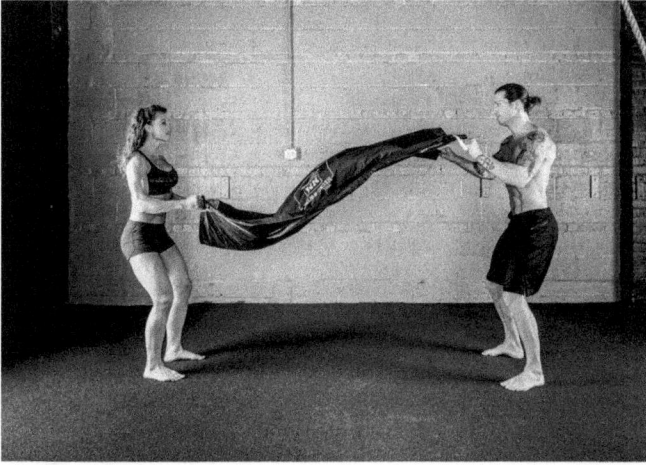

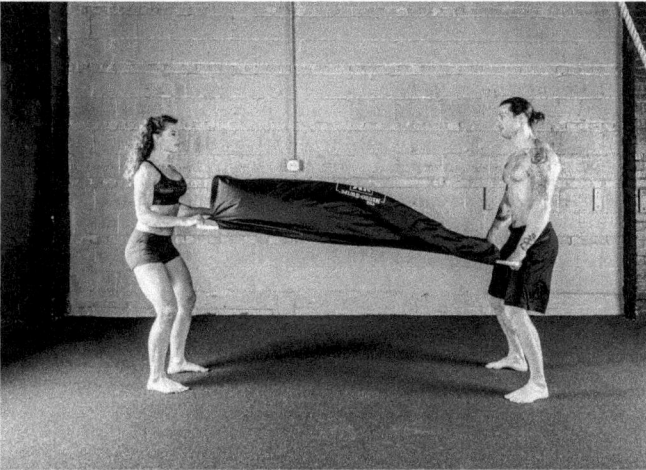

To vary the intensity of this foundational movement, adjust the distance the CCI travels up and down. Shortening the distance will ramp up the speed and heart rate. I find that the most effective range is from waist to shoulders.

I find that the most effective range is from waist to shoulders.

After you have mastered the velocity swipe, you are ready to begin the journey through the progressions and into Surge Sets.

The Exercises and Progressions

Commando Cardio incorporates an exceptional group of exercises that produce remarkable conditioning results. The exercises increase in difficulty and build upon one another. The progressions begin with exercises that focus on performing lower body isometrics and upper body dynamic movement at the same time. The advanced progressions will involve the lower body and upper body performing opposing dynamic movements simultaneously.

The exercises increase in difficulty and build upon one another.

This section will also include active recovery exercises that can be performed as a part of the Commando Cardio protocols. These drills will accelerate your results when used properly.

The standing overhand velocity swipe

Here is a quick review of the standing overhand swipe that is detailed in the previous chapter. Grasp the CCI with your palms facing down and pull them outward. Make sure you are the proper distance from your partner or anchor point. With the lower body tensed and the shoulders pulled down and back, begin to explosively drive the CCI upward. When the CCI reaches the eye level snap it back down forcefully. Do not let your hands drift inward. Repeat the movement creating as much speed as possible. Continue for 30 seconds.

The standing underhand velocity swipe

Once you have built the foundation with the standing overhand velocity swipe, you can now attempt the underhand version. Switching hand positions will change the upper body muscles that are targeted most. In the overhand version the shoulders, upper back, and trapezius muscles will fatigue quickly. In the overhand version the biceps, shoulders, chest and latissimus muscles receive a tremendous amount of work. It is essential to perform an equal amount of overhand and underhand conditioning to keep balanced development.

To begin, grasp the CCI with your palms facing upward and extend your hands outward. Your hands should be at waist level. Make sure that there is adequate distance between you and your partner or anchor point. Dig your toes into the ground and tighten your calf muscles. Keeping your knees slightly bent, tighten your quadriceps and hamstrings. Squeeze your gluteal muscles together until you feel a strong contraction. Do not hold your breath while getting the lower body set. Pull the shoulders back and down. Using the arms rapidly thrust the CCI upward until it reaches shoulder level. Immediately pull the CCI downward toward the ground. Continue this rapid up and down motion quickly and explosively for 15-30 seconds. Try to keep increasing the speed throughout the duration of the exercise.

Performance Points:

- Remember to keep the whole body engaged for the entire duration of the exercise.

- Fight the urge to slow down. The higher the velocity, the greater the conditioning effect.

- Do not let the hands slide inward, as this will decrease the resistance level.

- Don't allow your back and shoulders to round forward.

- Keep the shoulder blades pulled together.

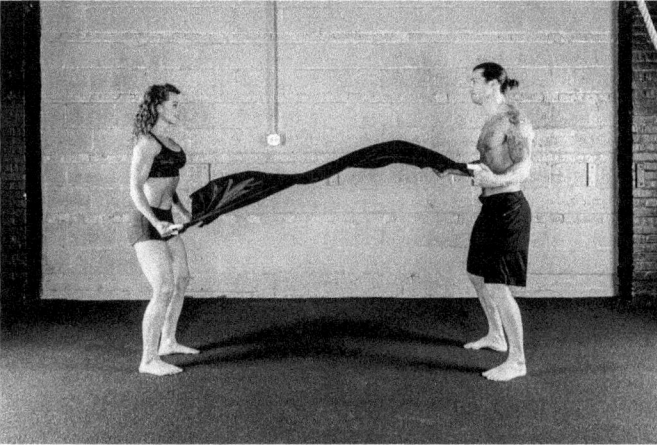

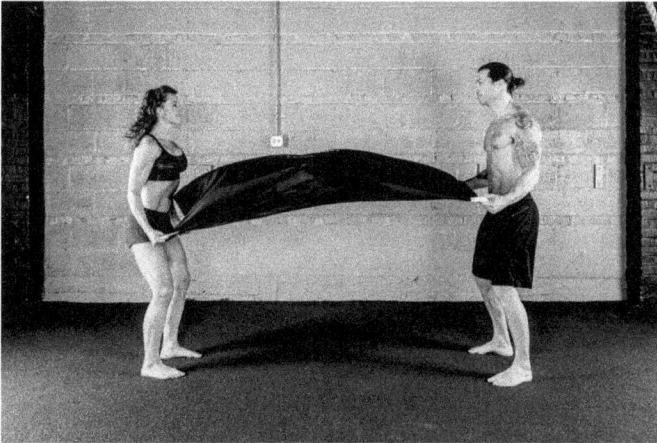

The lunging overhand velocity swipe

The lunge is one of the most common body positions found in sports. Being able to throw an implement or move weight rapidly from this position is a skill that is found in all elite athletes. Performing the overhand swipe while lunging is the next step in our progression of difficulty for many reasons. First of all, it challenges your ability to balance far more than standing. You will have to fight the urge to fall sideways; this brings the stabilizer muscles into play. This brings us to the second reason, the lunge's ability to tax the core. Holding a lunge isometrically requires a tremendous amount of core strength to keep the body upright and stabilized. A further reason is that it exposes muscle imbalances in the lower body. Where standing and squatting are lower body bilateral exercises, the lunge is unilateral. Many trainees find that when lunging, one side is stronger than the other. Regular use of this position will help identify these muscle imbalances and improve strength and performance. As a bonus, the lunging overhand swipe will improve flexibility by releasing tight hip flexors.

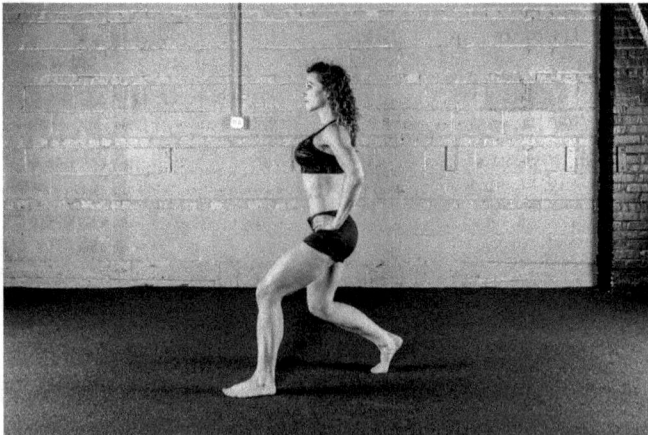

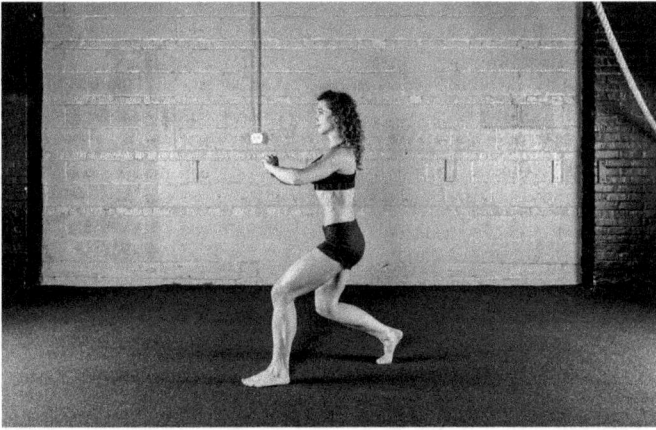

To begin, grasp the handles of the CCI in the overhand position and create the proper distance from your partner or anchor point. Now, step one foot behind you into a lunging position. The front foot should be in complete contact with the ground. The rear leg should be bent, and the knee should not be touching the floor. The toes of the rear foot should be in contact with the ground with the heel elevated. Digging the toes of the front foot into the ground, create tension in the calf muscle. Without moving your foot, drive your heel isometrically toward the rear leg. This should create tension in the hamstring and quadriceps. The toes of the rear leg should be spread and digging into the ground. Now isometrically drive the knee toward the ground. This should produce tension in the entire rear leg. You may want to practice getting into the position a few times before you add the upper body velocity motion.

Once you are in the correct isometric lunge position, spread the arms outward and pull the shoulder blades together. The hands should be at waist level. Now, explosively drive the CCI upwards until it reaches shoulder level. Immediately pull the CCI downward toward the ground. Continue this rapid up and down motion quickly and explosively for 15-30 seconds. Try to keep increasing the speed throughout the duration of the exercise. Work both legs equally.

Performance Points:

- Try to keep the back straight; do not lean forward.
- Do not lose tension in the lower body.
- Avoid twisting the upper body.
- Do not slow down.
- Do not allow the back and shoulders to round forward.

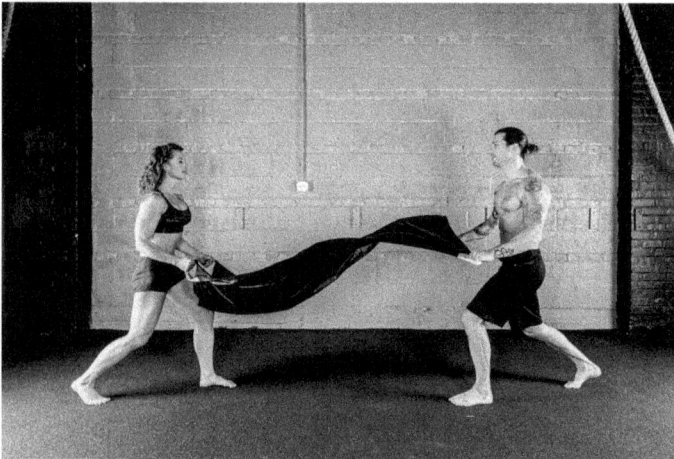

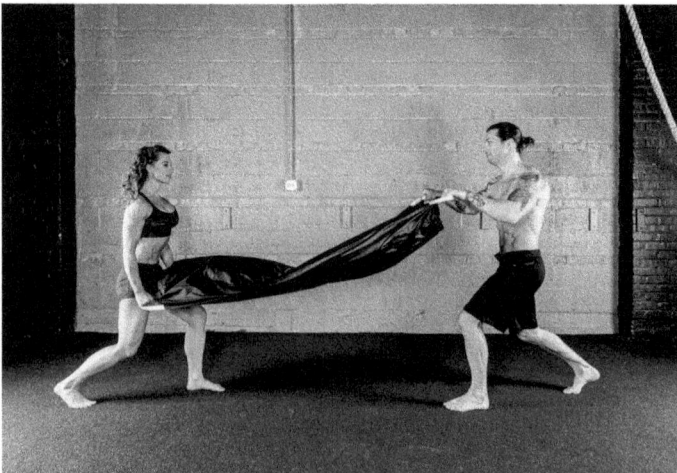

The lunging underhand velocity swipe

To perform the lunging underhand velocity swipe, grasp the handles of the CCI with your palms facing upward. Check to make sure that you have the proper distance between you and your partner or anchor point. Assume the same lower body position as in the previous exercise.

Make sure the hands are at waist level and the elbows are slightly bent. Pull the hands outward until the sides of the CCI are tight. Engage the scapula by pulling the shoulder blades together. Now, forcefully accelerate the CCI upwards until it reaches shoulder level. Immediately pull the CCI downward toward the ground. Continue this rapid up and down motion quickly and explosively for 15-30 seconds. Try to keep increasing the speed throughout the duration of the exercise. Work both legs equally.

Performance Points:

- Make sure you are not "curling" the CCI up and down.

- Focus on speed.

- Do not let your hands drift inward.

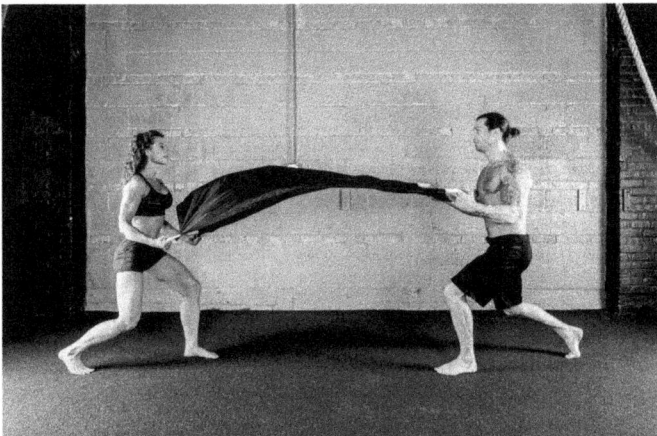

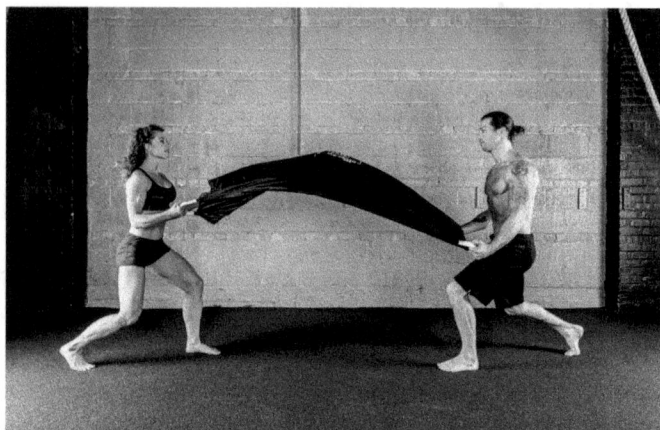

The squatting overhand velocity swipe

Squatting isometrically creates a strong base to support any athletic activity. The isometric squat builds powerful calves, hamstrings, quadriceps, glutes, and hips. The lower back and spinal erectors also receive a great amount of work. This exercise is also an excellent way to increase glute activation. When performed in an isometric fashion, it teaches the lower body to work together as unit.

An additional benefit of this lower body positioning is increased mobility. In the beginning, many trainees have a difficult time lowering into a full squat and holding it. Continued practice of this exercise leads to additional flexibility in the hips and groin. I have also found that the squatting overhand velocity swipe is an excellent tonic for the knees and ankles. The joints in the lower body will feel rejuvenated after performing Surge Sets in this position.

Start by grasping the CCI in the overhand position and establish the proper distance from your partner or anchor point. Place your feet shoulder width apart. Grip the ground with your toes and begin to actively pull yourself downward into the squat position. Focus on keeping the back straight as you are lowering.

Actively push the knees outward as you tense all the muscles in the lower body. Make sure to squeeze the glutes hard, as this will help keep proper positioning.

Once you are in the isometric squat, spread the arms outward and pull the shoulder blades together. The starting position for the hands depends on the depth the squat. The hands should start and finish high enough that they will not touch the legs. Using the arms, explosively drive the CCI upwards until it reaches shoulder level. Immediately pull the CCI downward toward the ground. The range of motion of the swipe is much smaller than in the previous positions. Continue this rapid up and down motion quickly and explosively for 15-30 seconds. Try to keep increasing the speed throughout the duration of the exercise.

Performance Points:

- Do not let the knees track inward; actively push them out.

- Keep your back as straight as possible.

- Do not "drop" into the position; rather, pull yourself down.

- Do not lose tension.

- Decrease the range of motion of the swipe.

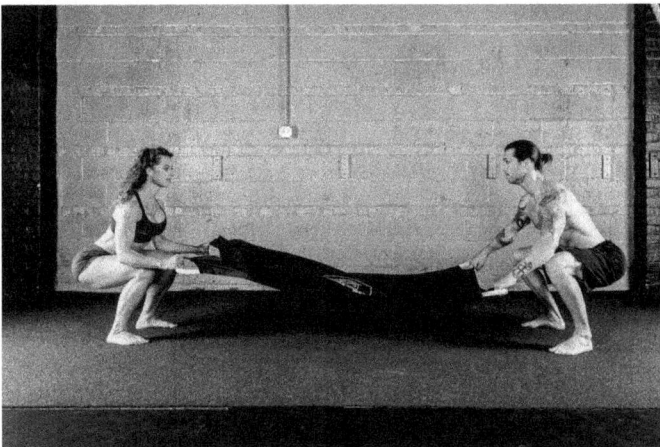

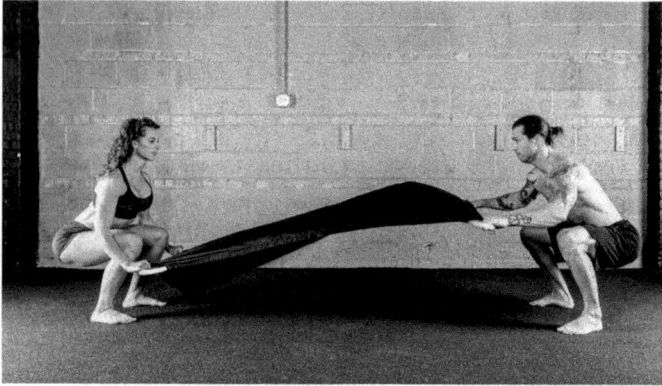

The squatting underhand velocity swipe

To perform the squatting underhand velocity swipe, place your hands on the CCI with your palms facing upward. Set the proper distance between you and your partner or anchor point. Assume the same lower body position as in the previous exercise. Make sure the hands are at a level higher than the knees. Pull the shoulder blades together and lower your shoulders. With the elbows slightly bent, explosively drive the CCI upwards until it reaches shoulder level. Immediately pull the CCI downward toward the ground. Remember the range of motion is short. Continue this rapid up and down motion quickly and explosively for 15-30 seconds. Try to keep increasing the speed throughout the duration of the exercise.

Performance Points:

- Don't hunch your shoulders upward.

- Fight the urge to lean forward.

- Keep tension on the entire lower body for the duration of the exercise.

- Avoid excessive bending at the elbows.

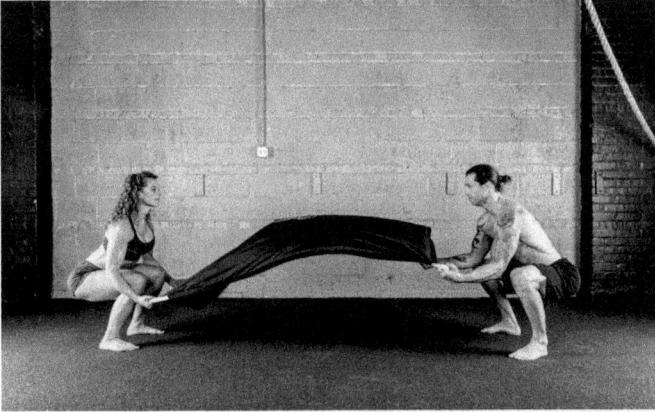

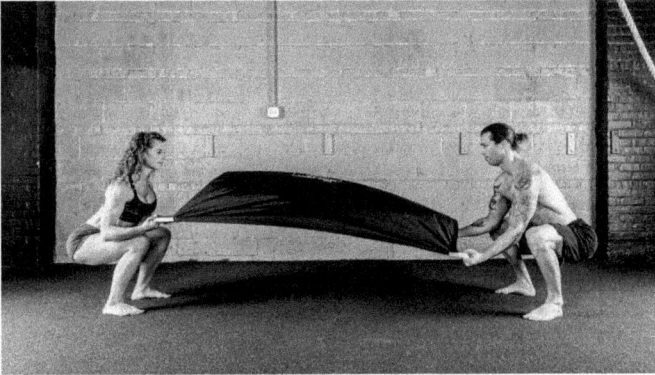

The kneeling overhand velocity swipe

The kneeling overhand swipe is more challenging because we are shortening the base. The base is the foundation for power production and by kneeling we increase the difficulty of the velocity swipe movement. You may want to have a mat or wear knee pads to protect knees. Even though you will be kneeling, the position is not passive; the lower body will still be activated isometrically.

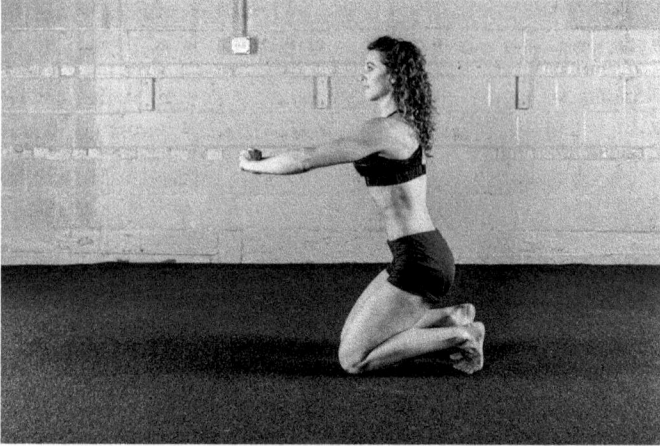

Begin by grasping the handles of the CCI in the overhand position and lower to your knees. Create the proper distance from your partner or anchor point. Push the ground away isometrically with the bottom of your toes, creating high tension in your calves. Now, move upward and begin flexing the quadriceps and hamstrings. Finally, tense the glutes hard.

Once you are in the correct isometric kneeling position, spread the arms outward and pull the shoulder blades together. The hands should be at waist level. Now, powerfully drive the CCI upwards until it reaches shoulder level. Immediately pull the CCI downward toward the ground. Continue this rapid up and down motion quickly and explosively for 15-30 seconds. Try to keep increasing the speed throughout the duration of the exercise.

Performance Points:

- Avoid excessive leaning backward.
- Avoid sitting on your heels.

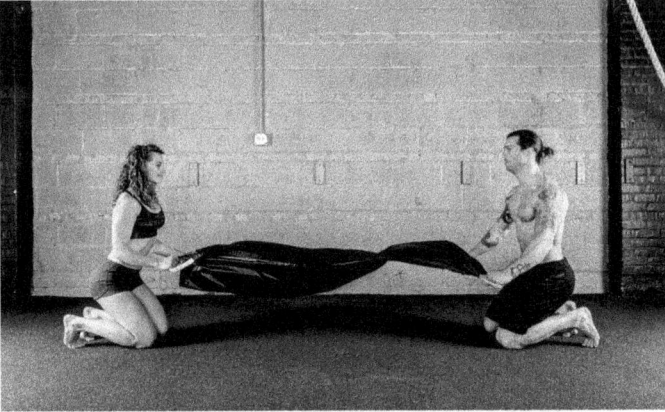

The kneeling underhand velocity swipe

Start by grasping the CCI with your palms facing upward. Get into the kneeling isometric position as in the previous exercise. Make sure there is adequate distance between you and your partner or anchor point. Extend the hands outward and slightly bend your elbows. Squeeze the shoulder blades together and keep the shoulders pulled downward. The hands should be at waist level. Now, powerfully drive the CCI upwards until it reaches shoulder level. Immediately pull the CCI downward toward the ground. Continue this rapid up and down motion quickly and explosively for 15-30 seconds. Try to keep increasing the speed throughout the duration of the exercise.

Performance Point: Avoid any bouncing motion from the knees. The goal is to keep the lower body contracted.

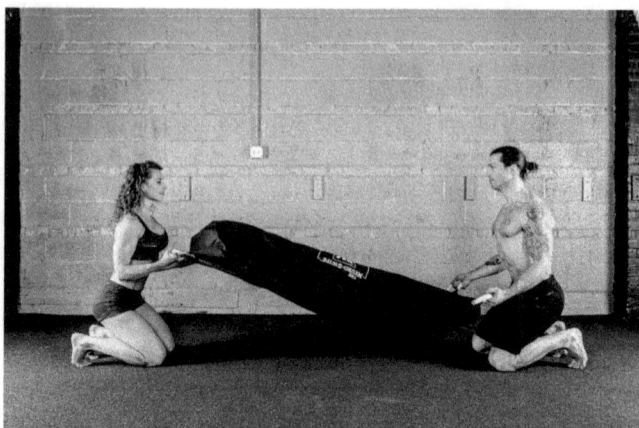
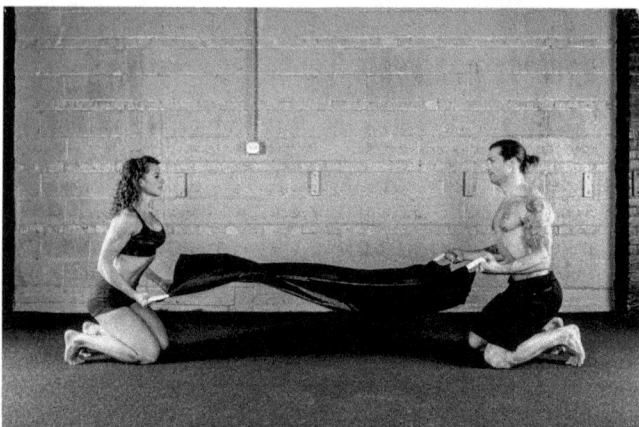
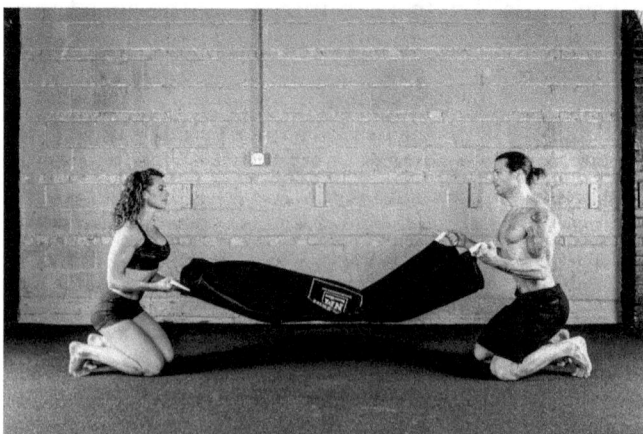

The V-straddle overhand velocity swipe

The next progression will challenge you in two ways: one, we are shortening the base even further and two, we are adding an isometric position that has a stretching component. Since all athletes have different levels of flexibility, the following position can be modified to accommodate your current capability.

Place the CCI on the ground in front of you. Sit down with your legs straightened and push them outward as far as possible. Now, dig your heels into the ground and isometrically try to pull your legs together. The toes should be pointed slightly outward. This isometric pull will create a large amount of tension the calves and hamstrings. Now, pull your kneecaps up and create tension in the quadriceps. Finally, squeeze the glutes hard.

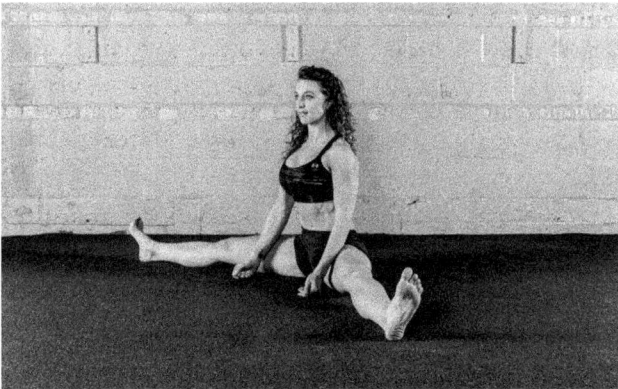

Now, pick up the CCI with an overhand grip. Spread the arms outward and pull the shoulder blades together. The starting position for the hands is just above the lower ribs. The hands should start and finish high enough that they will not touch the ground. Using the arms, explosively accelerate the CCI upwards until it reaches shoulder level. Immediately pull the CCI downward toward the ground. The range of motion of the swipe in this exercise is fairly short. Continue this rapid up and down motion quickly and explosively for 15-30 seconds. Try to keep increasing the speed throughout the duration of the exercise.

To modify this position, simply let your legs be placed closer together. Make sure to do the same isometric contraction as in the regular version. An advanced way to perform this exercise is to have a bar or some other object in between your feet to contract against. This will increase the isometric tension and flexibility in the lower body.

Performance Points:

- Do not round the back forward.

- Do not excessively lean backward.

- Because the range of the velocity swipe is small, you will have to increase the speed.

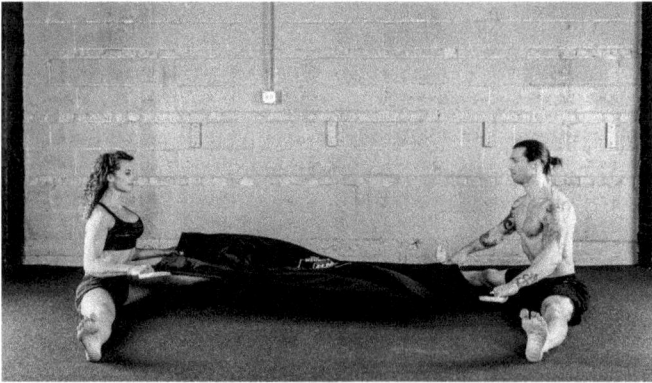

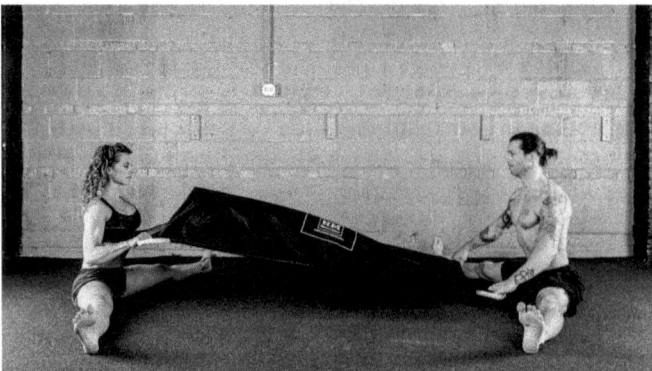

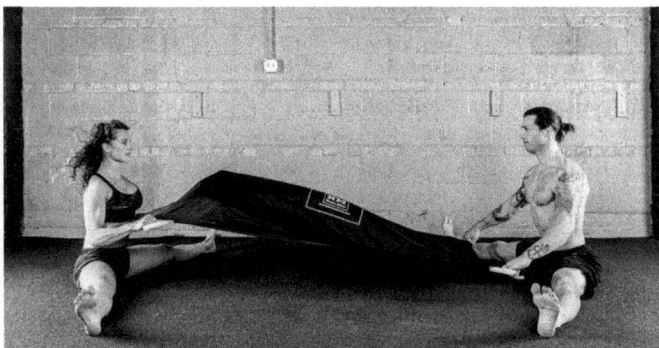

The V-straddle underhand velocity swipe

To perform the underhand version of this exercise, begin by getting into the V-straddle position. Now, grasp the CCI with an underhand grip. Spread the arms outward and pull the shoulder blades together. Make sure that the hands start and finish high enough that they will not touch the ground. With the elbows slightly bent, explosively drive the CCI upwards until it reaches shoulder level. Immediately pull the CCI downward toward the ground. Be aware that the range of motion in this version of the swipe is short. Continue this rapid up and down motion quickly and explosively for 15-30 seconds. Try to keep increasing the speed throughout the duration of the exercise.

Performance Point: Make sure that you are driving the CCI upward, not pulling it in toward you.

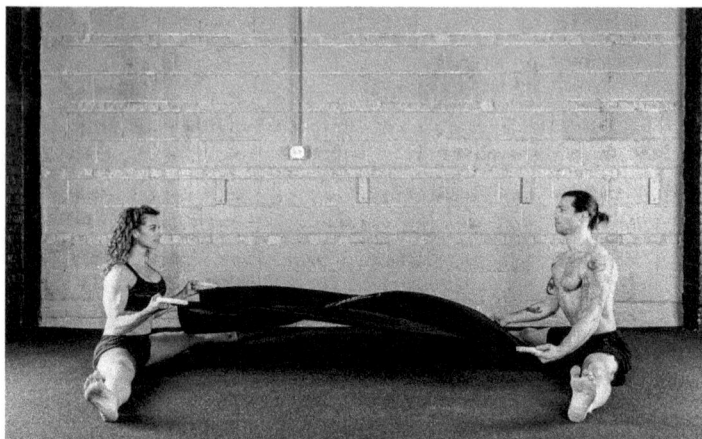
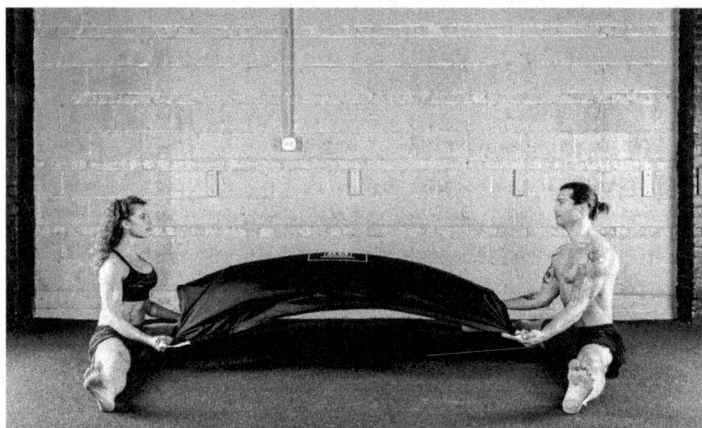
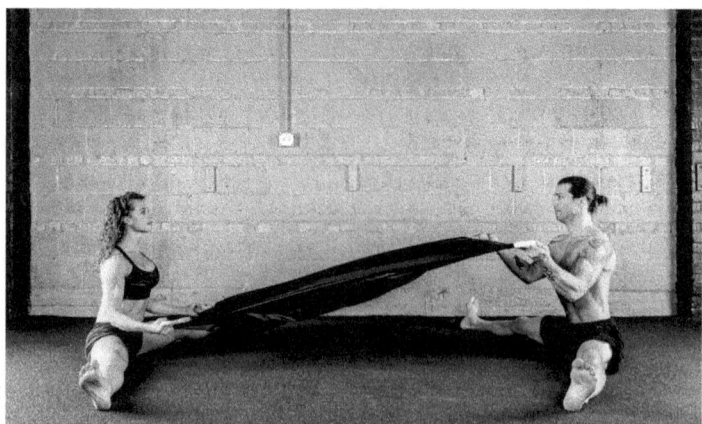

The front split overhand velocity swipe

This extreme progression of the velocity swipe should only be attempted if you are proficient in the front split. This exercise requires great flexibility and strength. To begin, assume the proper distance from your partner or anchor point and slowly lower into the front split position. Now, create tension in the lower body by driving the front heel and the back knee into the ground.

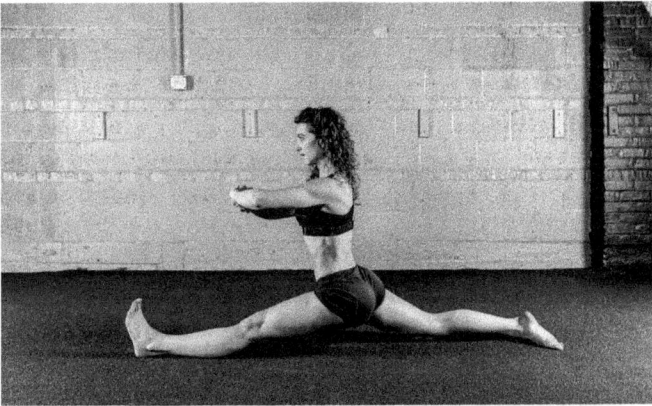

Once the lower body is properly positioned, grasp the CCI with the palms facing downward. Extend the hands outward and pull the shoulder blades together. The starting position for the hands is just above the lower ribs. Using the arms, explosively drive the CCI upwards until it reaches shoulder level. Immediately pull the CCI downward toward the ground. Performed correctly, the hands will start and finish high enough that they will not touch the legs. As in the previous exercise, the range of motion of the swipe is short. Continue this rapid up and down motion quickly and explosively for 15-30 seconds. Try to keep increasing the speed throughout the duration of the exercise.

Performance Points:

- If you are not proficient in the front split, this exercise is not for you!

- Remember to keep tension in the lower body for the duration of the entire exercise.

- Do not lean forward.

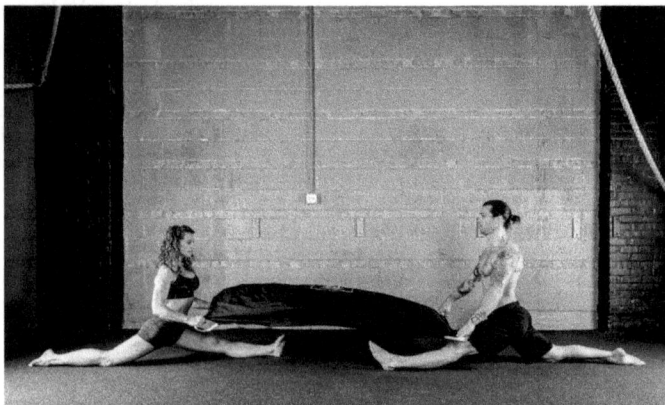

The front split underhand velocity swipe

After you have mastered the front split overhand velocity swipe, you are ready to progress to the underhand version. Establish the proper space between your partner or anchor point, and assume the front split position as in the previous exercise. Create tension by isometrically pushing the heel of the front foot and the knee of the back leg into the ground.

Now, grasp the CCI with the palms facing upward. With the elbows slightly flexed, extend the hands outward and pull the shoulder blades together. Position for the hands just above the lower ribs. Using the arms, explosively drive the CCI upwards until it reaches shoulder level. Immediately pull the CCI downward toward the ground. Make sure that the hands start and finish high enough that they will not touch the legs. Continue this rapid up and down motion quickly and explosively for 15-30 seconds. Try to keep increasing the speed throughout the duration of the exercise.

Performance Points:

- Do not excessively bend the elbows.

- Try to keep tension in the split for the duration of the exercise.

- Make sure to work both legs evenly.

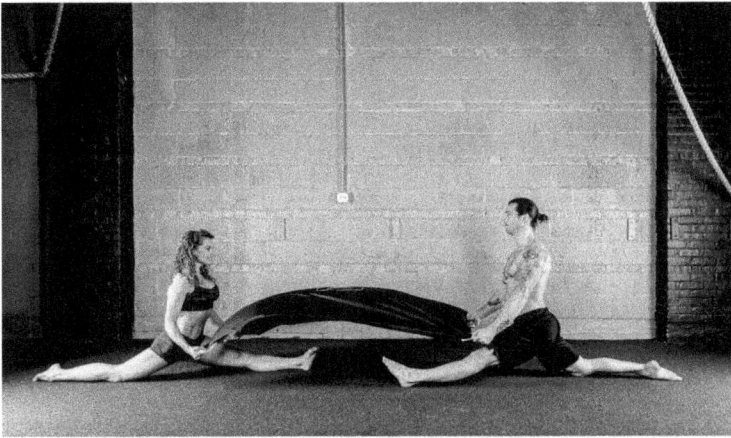

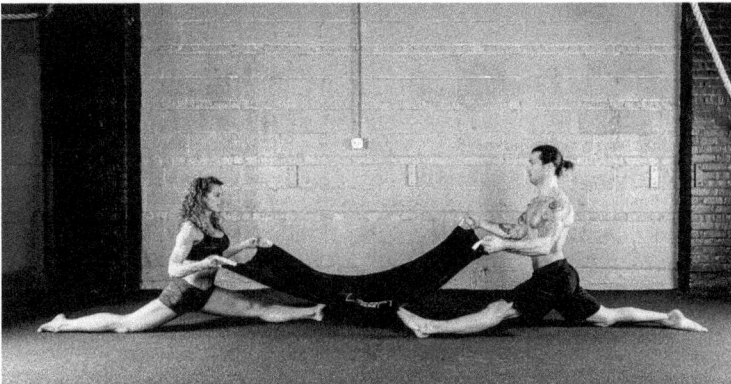

The scissors jump overhand velocity swipe combo

Before attempting the exercise combination, you should familiarize yourself with the scissors jump. The scissors jump will really work the quadriceps hard. Begin by placing the feet hip distance apart. Keeping the hips straight, step one foot backward and bend the knee. Now, forcefully jump into the air allowing both feet to change positions. When the feet make contact immediately repeat the movement. Practice the movement until you are comfortable performing it.

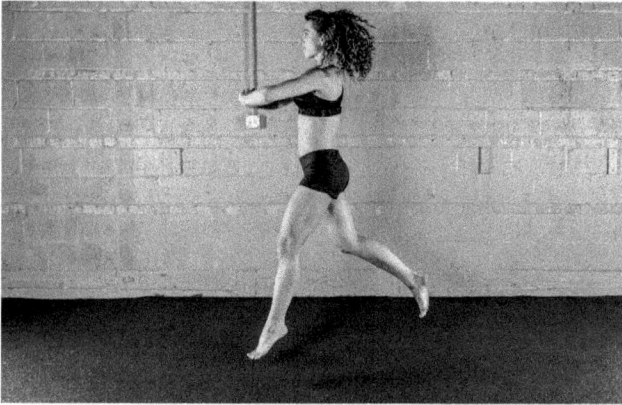

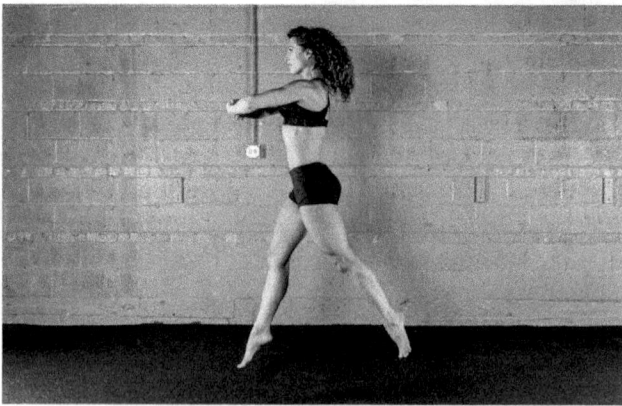

Now, you can add the velocity swipe to the scissor jump. Start by setting the proper distance from your partner or anchor point. Grasp the CCI with an overhand grip and spread the arms outward. Pull the shoulder blades together and step one foot backward into the beginning position for the scissor jump. Jump into the air, allowing the feet to change places while simultaneously accelerating the CCI up and down with the arms. The range of motion for arms should be waist to shoulder. The speed of the velocity swipe should be faster the scissor jumps. Keep performing this jumping and swiping combination for 15-30 seconds.

Performance Point: Keep the swipe motion faster than the scissor jumps.

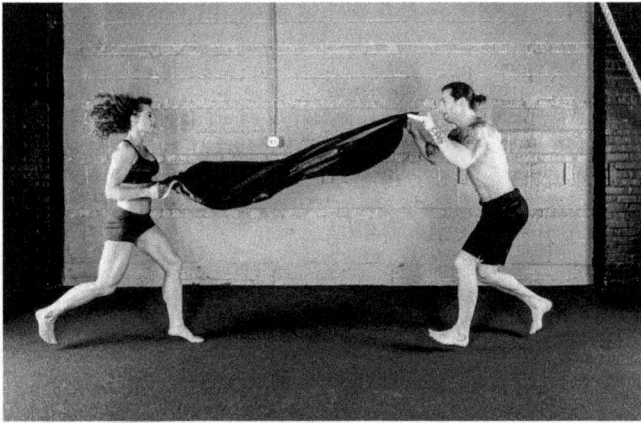

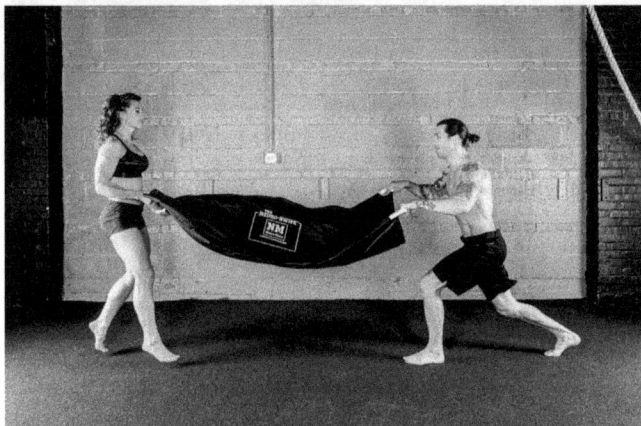

The scissors jump underhand velocity swipe combo

Begin by assuming the appropriate distance from your partner or anchor point. Pick up the CCI and grip with the palms facing upward. With elbows slightly bent, move the arms outward and pull the shoulder blades together. Set one foot backward until you are in the beginning position for the scissors jump. Now, jump into the air allowing the feet to change places while simultaneously driving the CCI up and down with arms. The range of motion for arms should be waist to shoulder. The speed of the velocity swipe should be faster the scissors jumps. Keep performing this jumping and swiping combination for 15-30 seconds.

Performance Point: Keep the swipe motion faster than the scissor jumps.

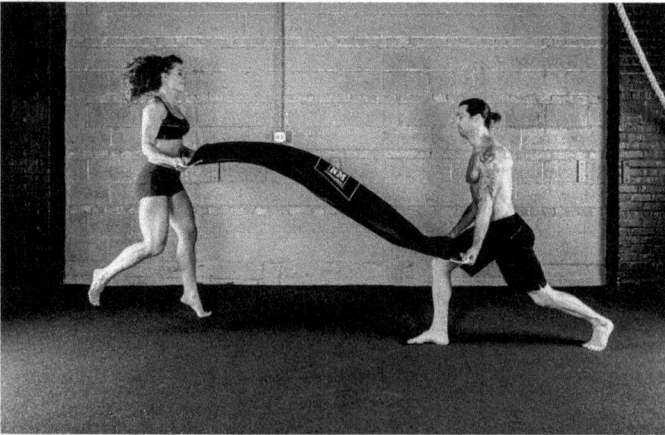

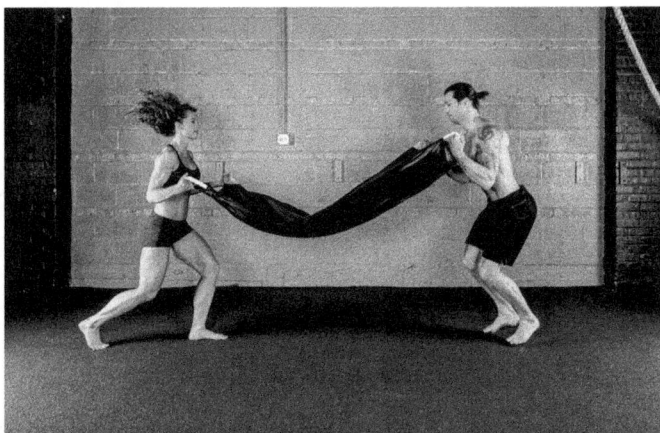

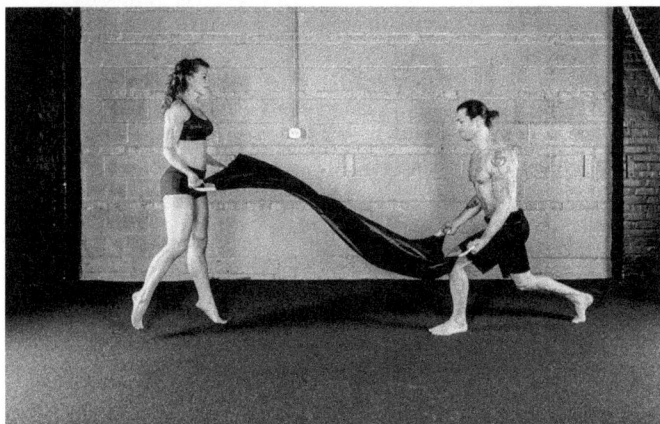

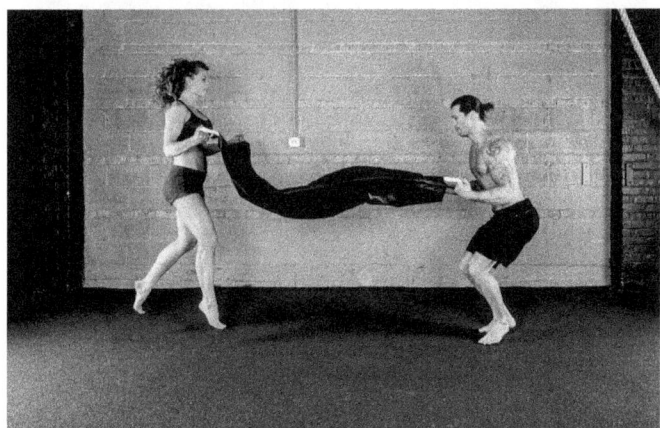

The criss-cross jump overhand velocity swipe combo

It would be wise to master the basic criss-cross jump before attempting the combo. This exercise will be very taxing on your quadriceps, glutes, inner thighs, and abdominals. It will also challenge your coordination. To begin, place your feet shoulder width apart. Bend the knees slightly and bring the heels about one inch off the floor. The leg motion is the same as a jumping jack except that you are going to allow the feet to continue past the normal stopping point until they cross over each other. Jump upwards until the legs cross and upon landing immediately reverse the movement. Continue jumping alternating the forward leg.

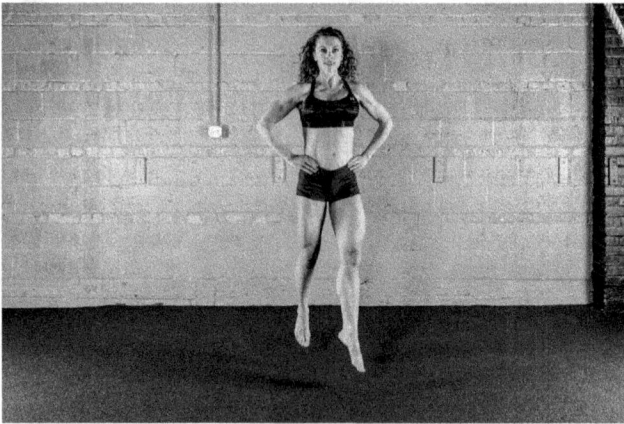

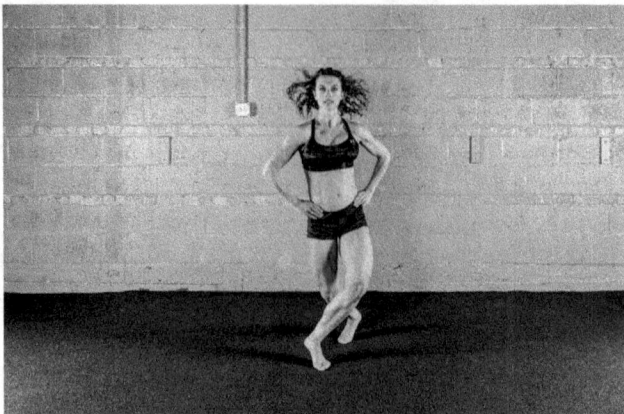

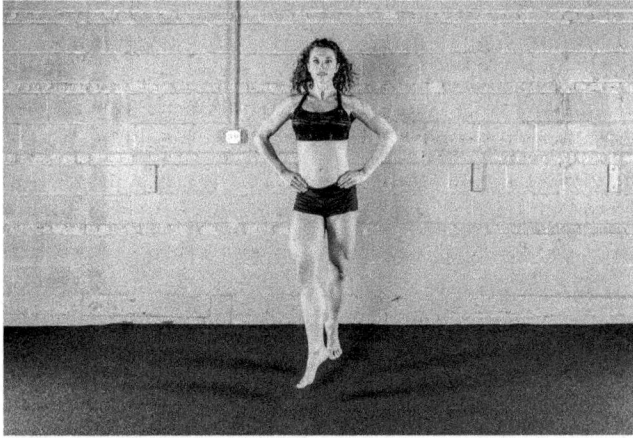

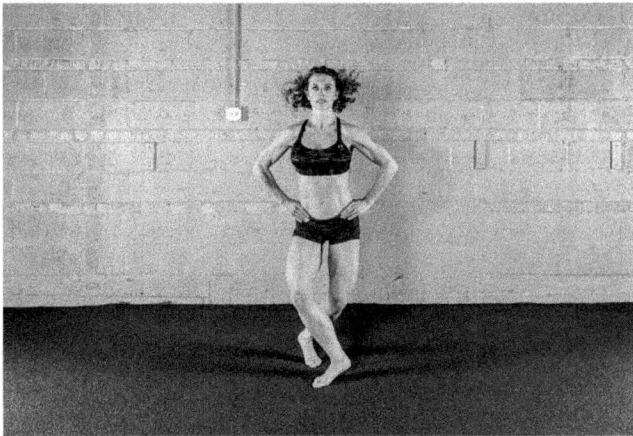

After you have had a chance to practice the criss-cross jump, you can add the velocity swipe to the exercise. Begin by setting the proper distance from your partner or anchor point. Grasp the CCI with an overhand grip and spread the arms outward. Pull the shoulder blades together and assume the beginning position for the criss-cross jump. Jump into the air, allowing the feet to cross while simultaneously accelerating the CCI up and down with arms. The range of motion for arms should be waist to shoulder. The speed of the velocity swipe should be faster the criss-cross jumps. Keep performing this jumping and swiping combination for 15-30 seconds.

Performance Point: Keep the swipe motion moving faster than the criss-cross jumps.

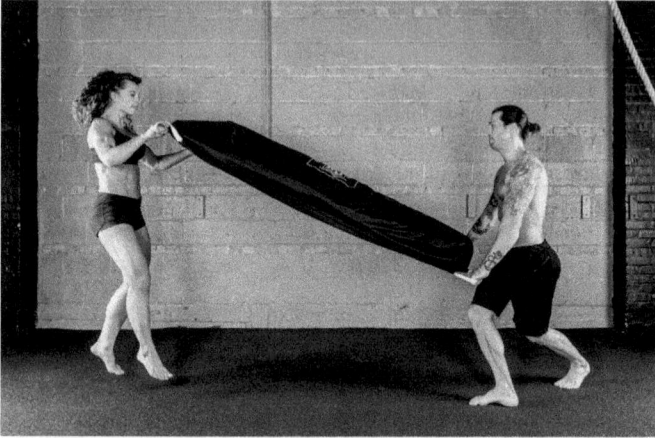

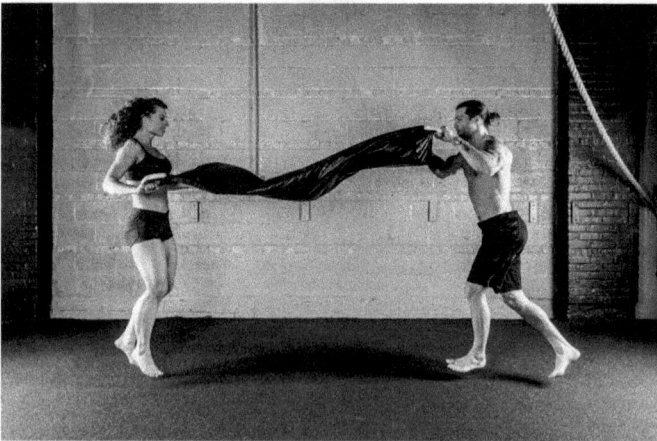

The criss-cross jump underhand velocity swipe combo

To perform the criss-cross jump underhand velocity swipe combo, create the proper distance from your partner or anchor point. Now, grasp the CCI with the palms facing upward. With elbows slightly bent, move the arms outward and pull the shoulder blades together. Set the lower body into the beginning position for the criss-cross jump. Now, jump into the air allowing the feet to cross one another while simultaneously driving the CCI up and down with arms. The range of motion for arms should be waist to shoulder. The speed of the velocity swipe should be faster the criss-cross jumps. Keep performing this jumping and swiping combination for 15-30 seconds.

Performance Point: Keep the swipe motion moving faster than the criss-cross jumps.

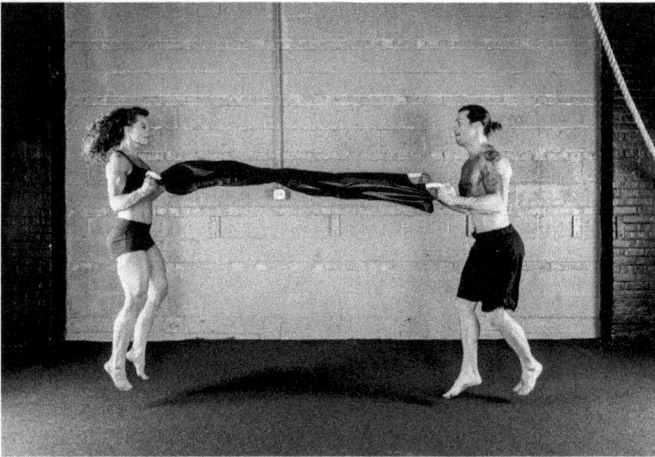

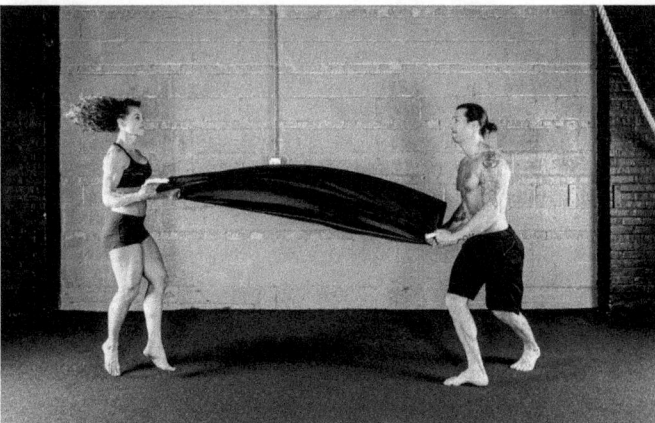

The jump squat overhand velocity swipe combo

Before attempting this exercise combination, make sure you are able to perform the jump squat correctly. The jump squat builds tremendous power and strength. Start by setting your feet shoulder width apart and pulling yourself down into a low squat position. When you reach the desired depth, drive your feet through the ground and accelerate upward until the body is airborne. Make sure that you land on the balls of your feet and repeat the movement.

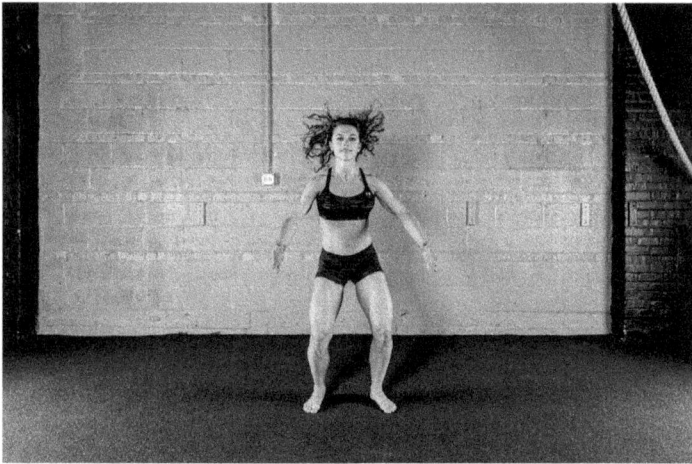

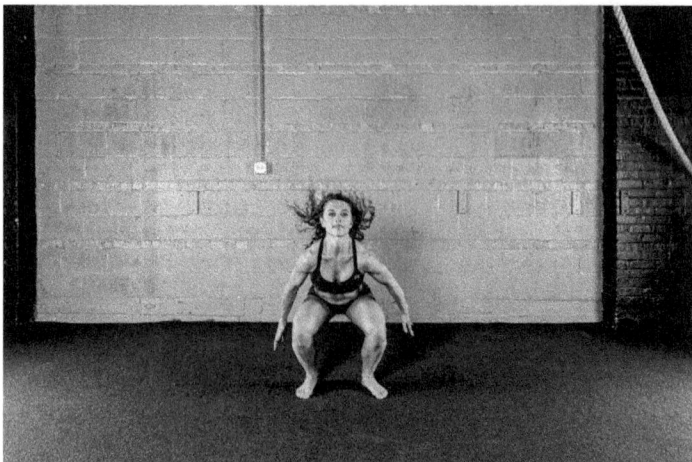

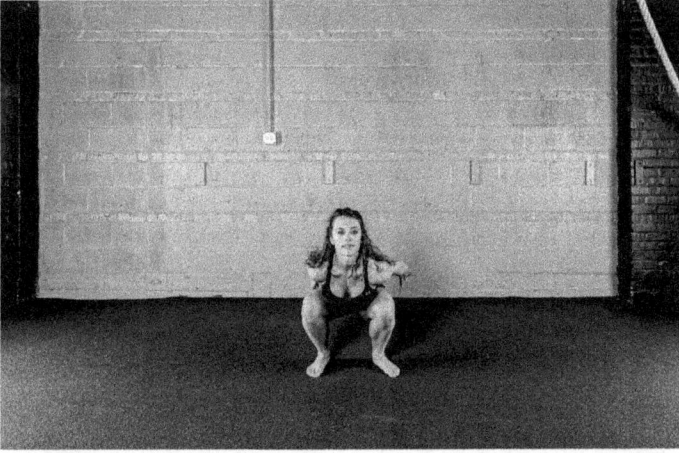

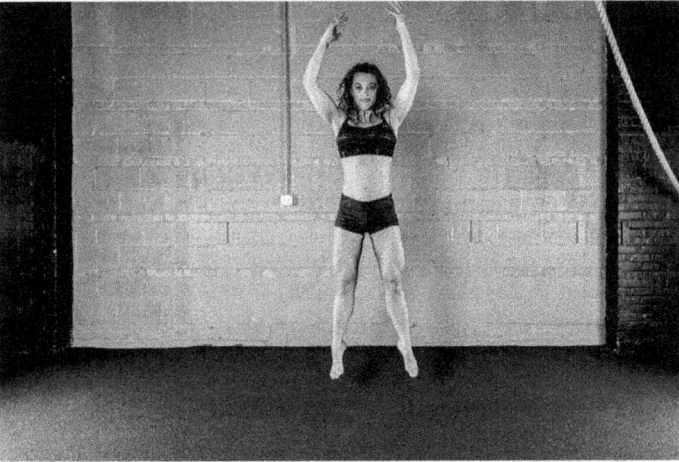

After you have spent some time working on the jump squat, you can add the velocity swipe to the exercise. Begin by setting the proper distance from your partner or anchor point. Grasp the CCI with an overhand grip and spread the arms outward. Pull the shoulder blades together and position your feet shoulder width apart. Squat down and explosively jump into the air allowing the feet to leave the ground while simultaneously driving the CCI up and down with arms. The range of motion for arms should be waist to shoulder. Try to coordinate the timing of the jumps to be in sync with your partner. Another variation is allowing one partner to start in the squat while the other is standing. This produces a see-saw jumping effect. The speed of the velocity swipe should be faster the jump squats. Keep performing this jumping and swiping combination for 15-30 seconds.

Performance Point: Always keep the speed of the swipe movement faster than the jump squats.

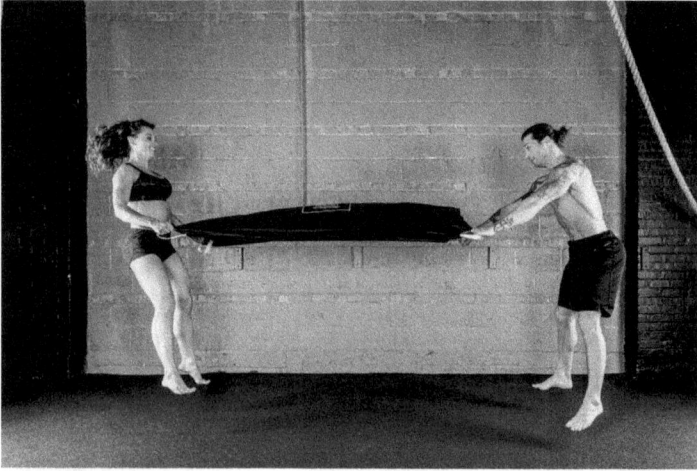

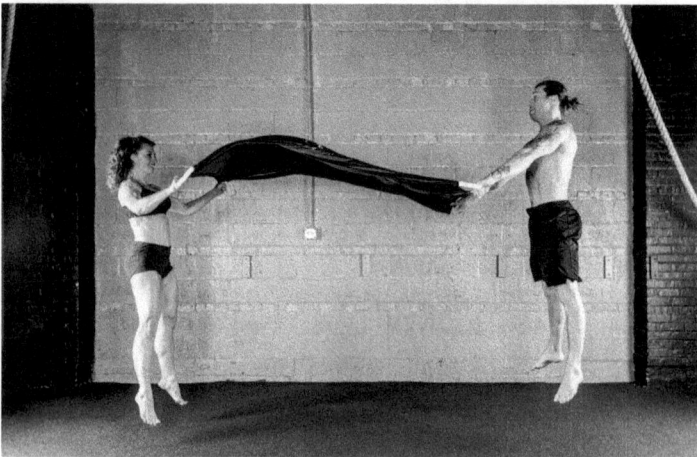

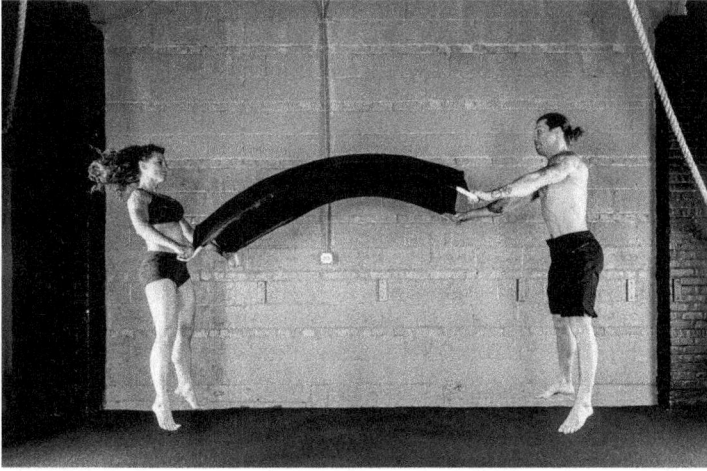

The jump squat underhand velocity swipe combo

Begin by creating the appropriate distance from your partner or anchor point. Pick up the CCI with the palms facing upward. With elbows slightly bent, move the arms outward and pull the shoulder blades together. Set the feet shoulder width apart. Now, drop into a deep squat and then jump explosively into the air while simultaneously driving the CCI up and down with arms. The range of motion for your arms should be waist to shoulder. As in the previous combination, try to time the jumps with your partner or attempt the see-saw variation. The speed of the velocity swipe should be faster the jump squats. Keep performing this jumping and swiping combination for 15-30 seconds.

Performance Point: Always keep the speed of the swipe movement faster than the jump squats.

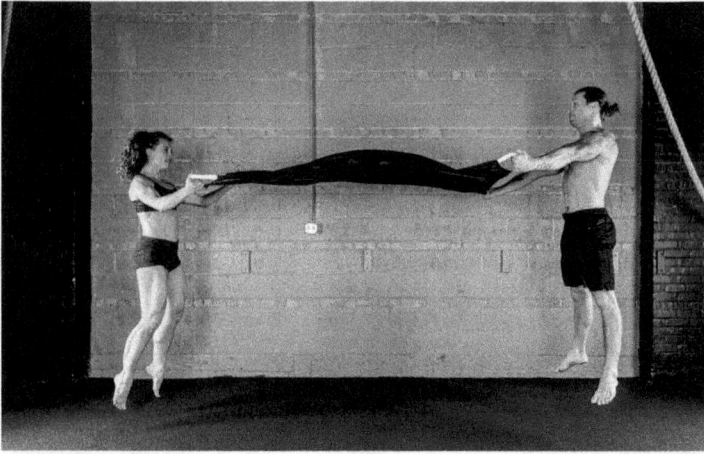

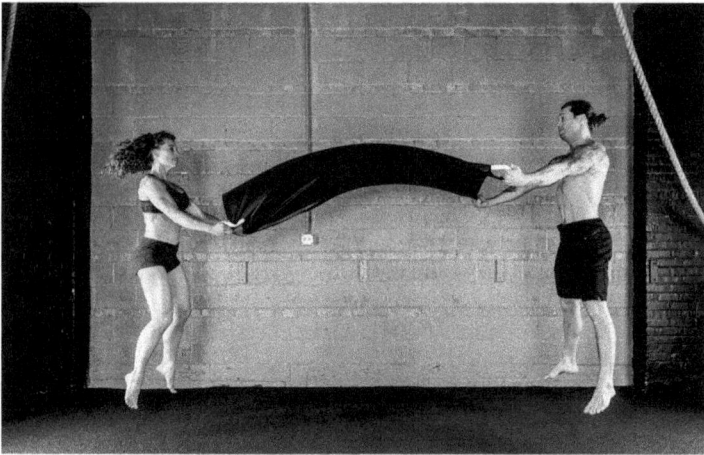

The lateral shuffle overhand velocity swipe combo

The ability to change directions laterally is a coveted skill for all athletes. The lateral shuffle overhand velocity swipe will improve agility and athleticism when practiced regularly. This exercise is best performed with a partner. Another benefit from this drill is learning to mirror your partner's lateral movement. This is a great benefit for those who compete in sports and must defend or guard against another athlete.

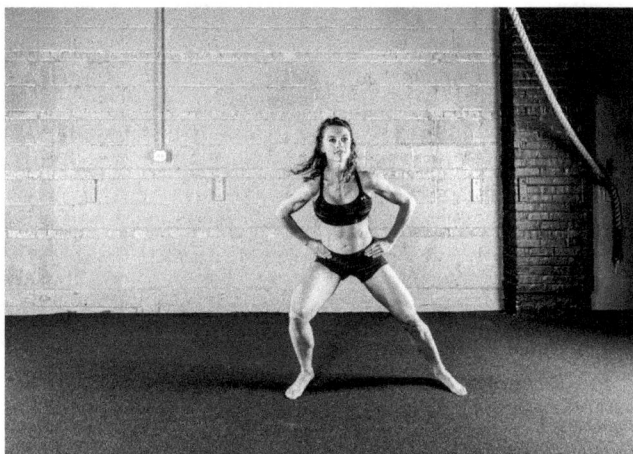

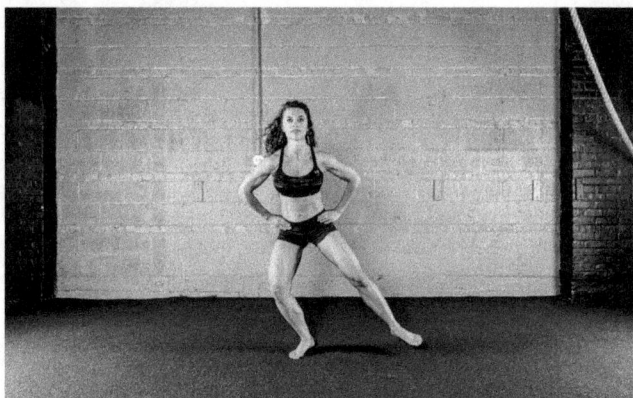

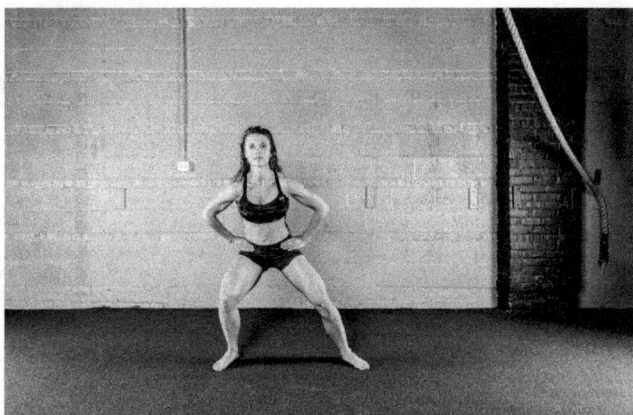

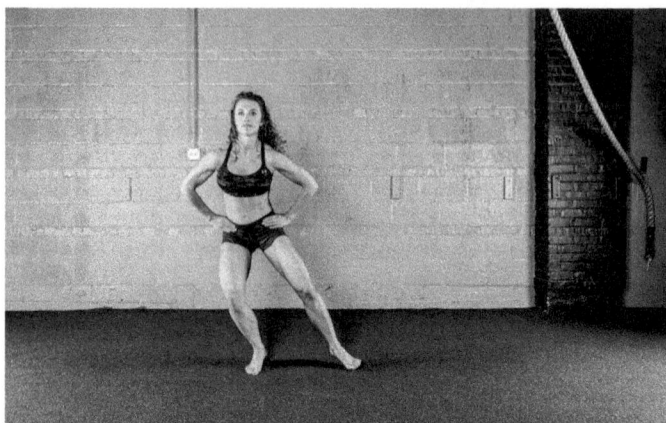

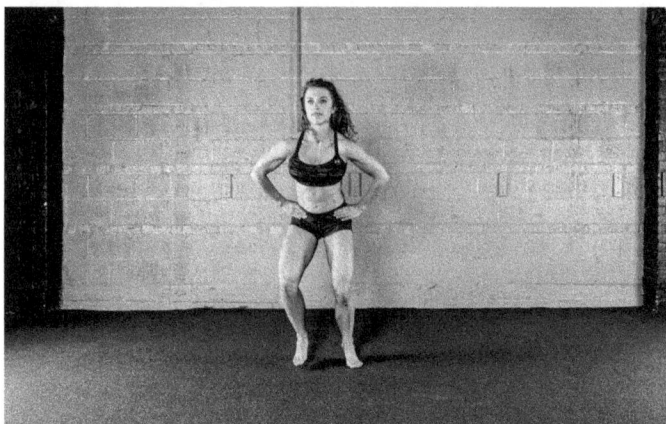

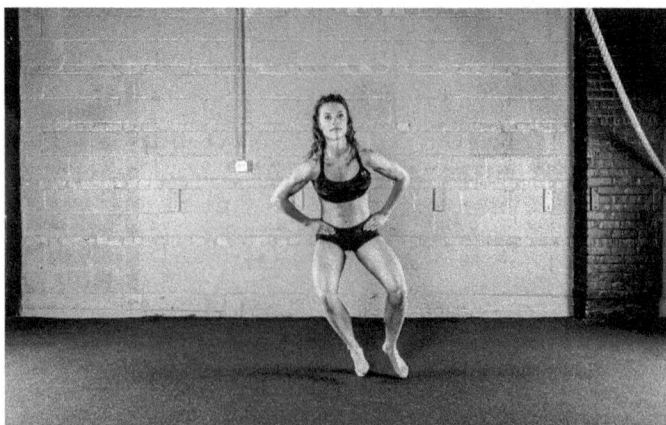

Start by assuming the proper distance from your partner. Grasp the CCI with an overhand grip and spread the arms outward. Pull the shoulder blades together and position your feet shoulder width apart. Let the lower body drop into a quarter squat. Allow one partner to call the lateral direction that you will be moving toward. Pushing off the trailing foot, explode laterally while allowing the lead foot to become airborne. Once the lead foot reaches the ground, push off it to continue the lateral movement. As the lower body is moving, the CCI should be accelerating up and down with arms. The range of motion for arms should be waist to shoulder. Alternate which partner is calling the directional shift. The speed of the velocity swipe should be faster than the lateral shuffle. Keep performing this shuffling and swiping combination for 15-30 seconds.

Performance Point: Increase the difficulty of the movement by using random distances when calling for a change in direction. This challenges your partner by trying to catch them "off-guard" during the performance of the exercise.

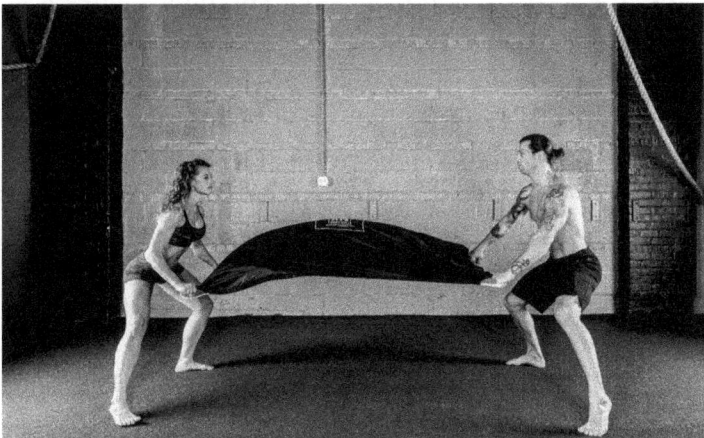

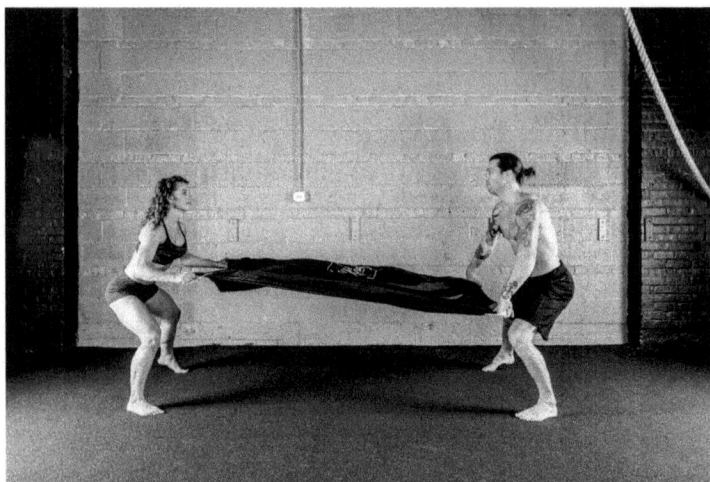

The lateral shuffle underhand velocity swipe combo

To perform the lateral shuffle underhand velocity swipe combo, create the proper distance from your partner. Now, grasp the CCI with the palms facing upward. With elbows slightly bent, move the arms outward and pull the shoulder blades together. Set the lower body into a quarter squat, which is the beginning position for the lateral shuffle. Decide which partner will call the first lateral direction that you will be moving. Push off the trail foot, and explode laterally while allowing the lead foot to become airborne. Once the lead foot reaches the ground, push off it to continue the lateral movement. As the lower body is moving laterally, simultaneously drive the CCI up and down with arms. The range of motion for arms should be waist to shoulder. Alternate which partner is calling the directional shift. The speed of the velocity swipe should be faster than the lateral shuffle. Keep performing this shuffling and swiping combination for 15-30 seconds.

Performance Point: Increase the difficulty of the movement by using random distances when calling for a change in direction.

This challenges your partner by trying to catch them "off-guard" during the performance of the exercise.

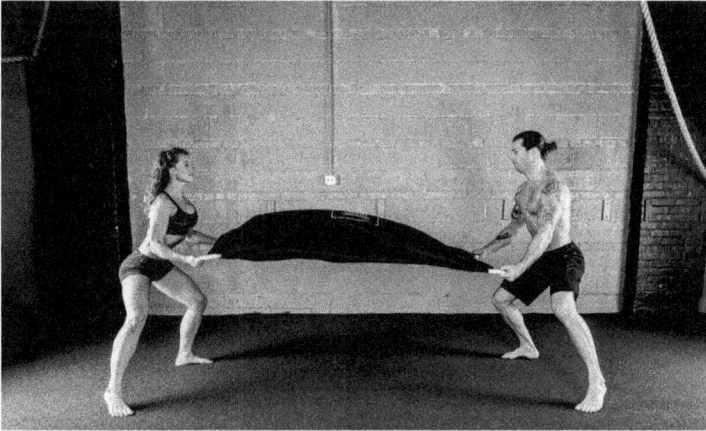

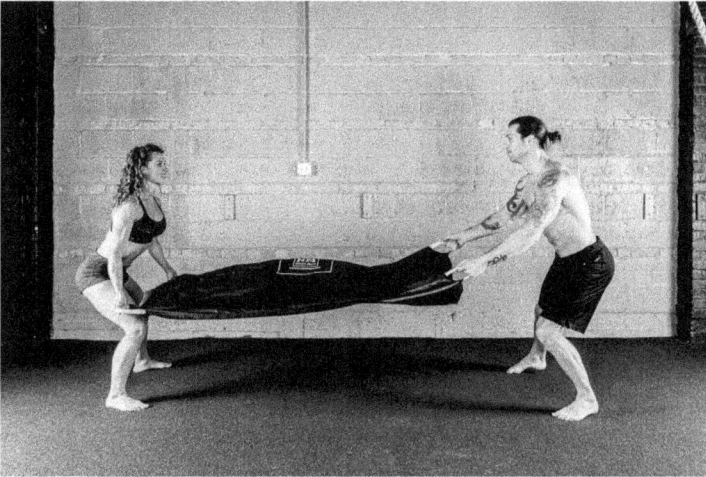

The lateral hop overhand velocity swipe combo

Before attempting this exercise combination, you should familiarize yourself with the lateral hop. The lateral hop will develop balance, strength, coordination, and the stabilizer muscles in the lateral chain. This exercise will download the skill of being able to make a cut, juke, or explosively change directions on the field and court. Begin by placing an object like a rolled-up towel on the outside of one of your feet. Now, squat downward and explosively launch your body laterally over the object while pulling your knees in toward your chest. After your feet touch the ground, forcefully launch in the other direction over the object. Continue repeating the jumping movement. Practice this exercise until you are comfortable performing it.

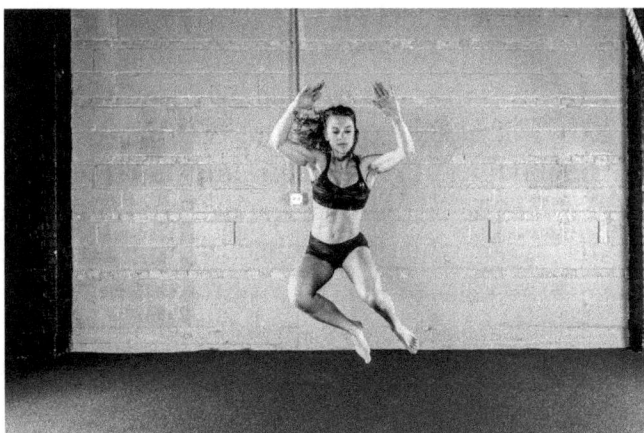

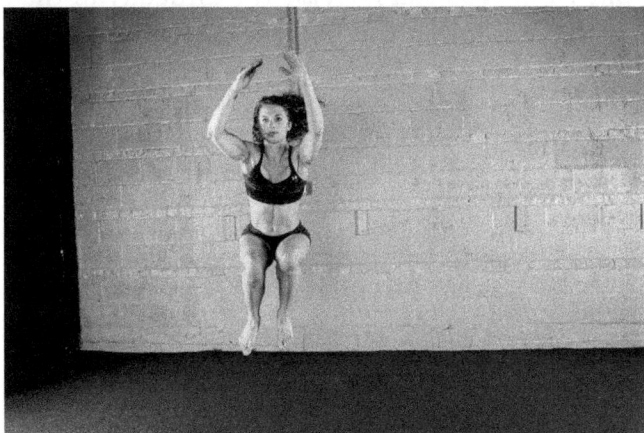

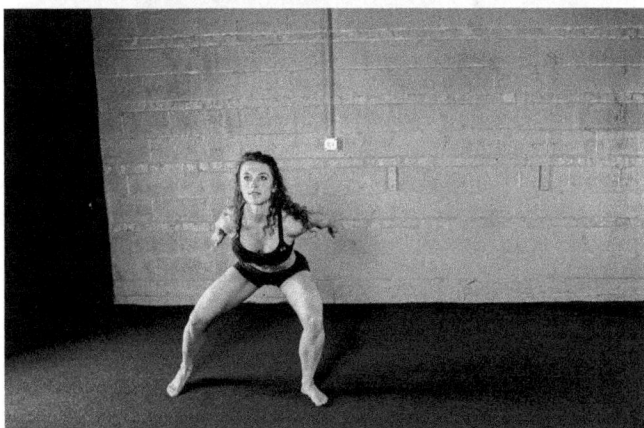

After you have mastered the lateral hop, you are ready to perform the combination. Start by setting the proper distance from your partner. Grasp the CCI with an overhand grip and spread the arms outward. Decide which direction you will start with. Now, pull the shoulder blades together and lower into the beginning position for the lateral hop. Launch yourself upward and laterally into the air while simultaneously driving the CCI up and down with the arms. The range of motion for arms should be waist to shoulder. Make sure the hops are in sync with your partner. Keep performing this jumping and swiping combination for 15-30 seconds.

Performance Point: You can increase the difficulty of the exercise by making the object that you hop over higher or wider.

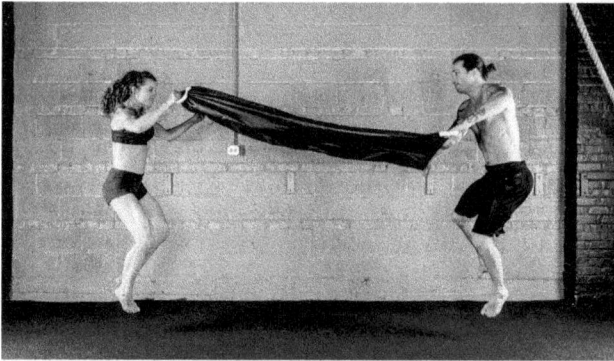

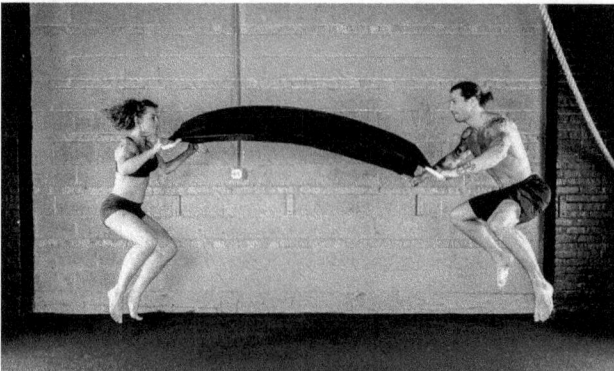

The lateral hop underhand velocity swipe combo

To perform the lateral hop underhand velocity swipe combo, create the proper distance from your partner. Now, grasp the CCI with the palms facing upward. With elbows slightly bent, move the arms outward and pull the shoulder blades together. Set the lower body into the beginning position for the lateral hop. Now, launch laterally into the air allowing the knees to come in towards the chest while simultaneously accelerating the CCI up and down with arms. The range of motion for arms should be waist to shoulder. Make sure the jumps are timed correctly with your partner. Keep performing this jumping and swiping combination for 15-30 seconds.

Performance Point: You can increase the difficulty of the exercise by making the object that you hop over higher or wider.

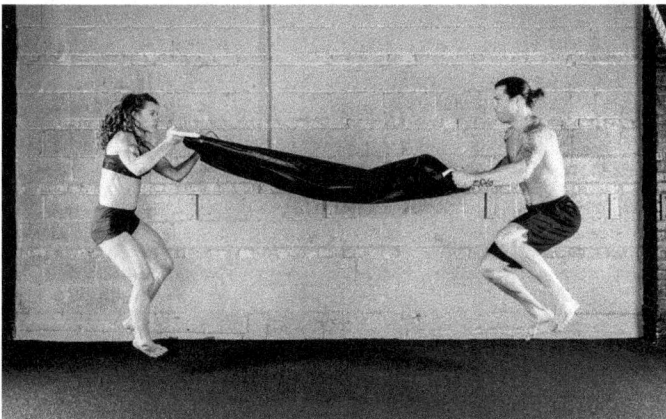

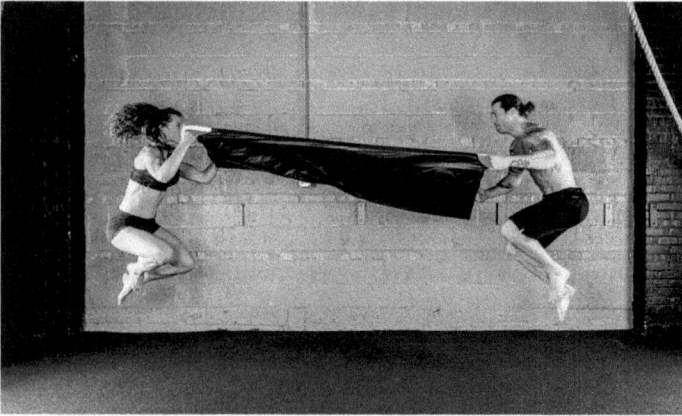

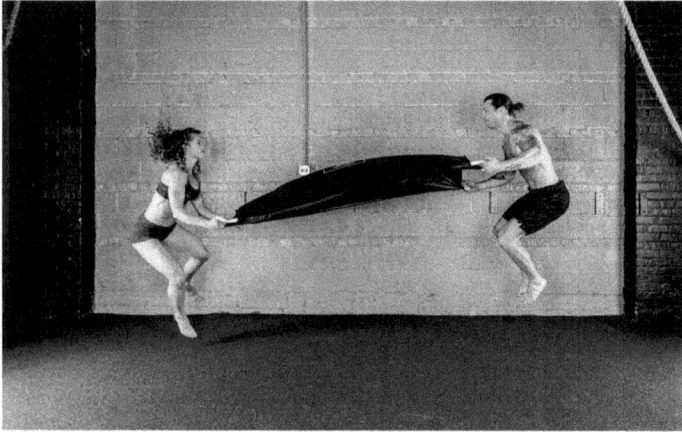

Increase the effectiveness of your Surge Sets with "resistance recovery"

After performing a Surge Set, there is a time for rest or recovery. Resistance recovery is just what the name suggests. Instead of traditional rest between sets, you will perform light resistance exercises that will increase the overall effectiveness of the Commando Cardio program.

Resistance recovery keeps the body primed for action. By continuing to move during recovery periods, we are sending signals throughout the entire body that the workout is not over. This also keeps the muscles warm and helps to alleviate the shock to the system that occurs when there is a sudden complete stop during intense training.

Resistance recovery keeps the body primed for action.

Resistance recovery also helps to remove the lactic acid from the musculature, so you can give an all-out effort on each Surge Set. These drills assist in flushing waste out of the system while keeping a steady blood flow to the muscles. This means that you will feel fresher and be able to perform harder and longer.

These drills also help to keep proper body symmetry. This is accomplished by performing light resistance pulls and extensions to balance out the high speed up and down swiping motion.

The key is to perform the exercises at a low intensity/ resistance level. Too much exercise during the rest period = no recovery.

Biceps pull resistance recovery drill

To perform this drill, grasp the CCI with your palms facing upward. Bring your arms upward until your arms are parallel to the floor. Now, allow one partner to pull the CCI in towards the upper body by bending the elbows until the forearms and biceps form a 90-degree angle. The other partner should step backward keeping their arms straight until the CCI is taut.

This is the starting position for the bicep pull. The partner with straight arms should now begin to pull the CCI toward the upper body, while the other partner provides light assistance. Once the forearm and bicep form a 90-degree angle, reverse the movement. Continue this back and forth motion for 15-30 seconds. The positive and negative resistance on the biceps make this an excellent recovery drill.

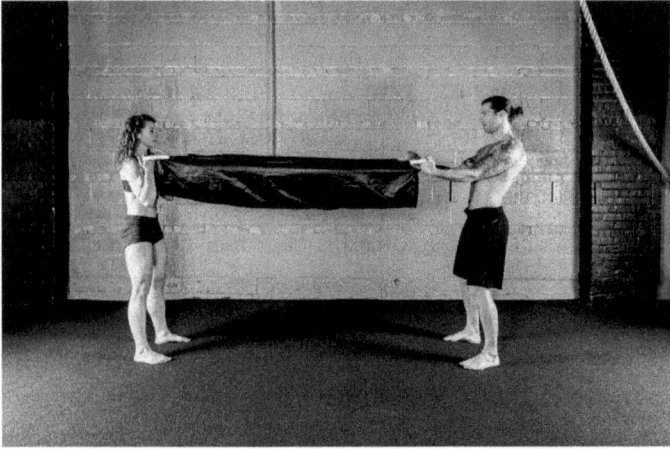

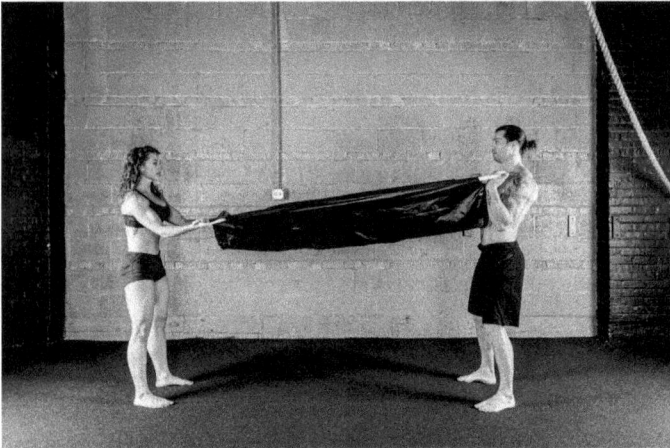

Triceps extension resistance recovery drill

Getting into the beginning position for this drill is more challenging than the others, but it is worth the effort. Begin by having both partners facing each other and grasping the CCI with an overhand grip. Now, bring the arms to one side and continue upwards while rotating the body until both partner's backs are facing each other with the arms overhead. Now, allow one partner to bend at the elbows bring the hands downward toward the shoulders. The other partner should keep the arms straight over the head and step the proper distance until the CCI is taut. This is the beginning position for the drill. The partner with bent arms should now begin to pull their arms upward while the other partner allows the arms to move toward the shoulders. Provide light partner resistance and continue the movement back and forth for 15-30 seconds. This drill gives a great stretch to the triceps and latissimus muscles.

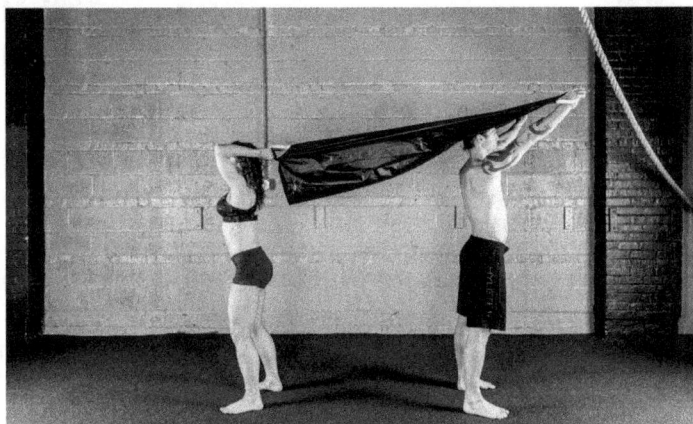

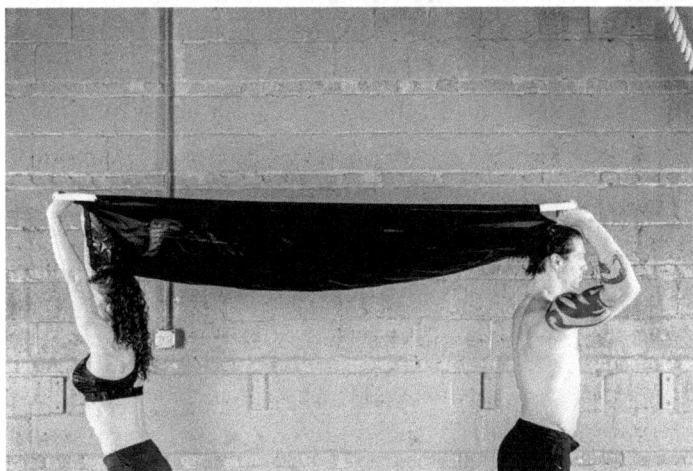

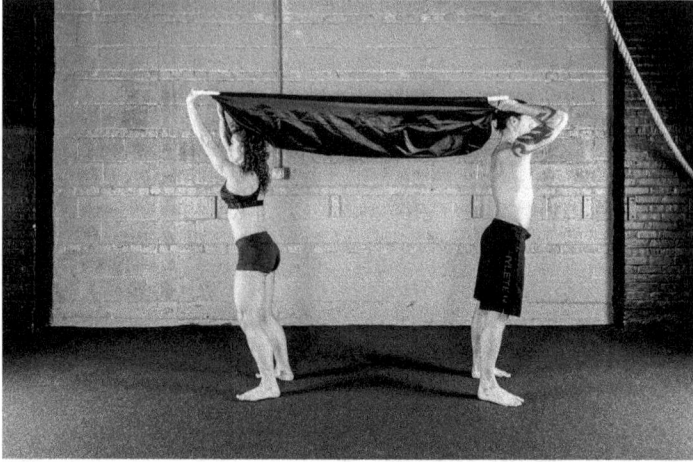

Row pull resistance recovery drill

This is my personal favorite resistance recovery drill. Begin by grasping the CCI in an overhand grip. Have one partner pull the CCI toward the chest with a rowing motion. As the hands come toward the chest, allow the wrists to rotate until they are facing one another. The other partner should keep the arms straight and step back until the CCI is taught. This is the beginning position for the drill. Now, the partner with straight arms should begin to pull the CCI toward the chest with a rowing motion allowing the wrists to rotate until they are facing one another. Reverse the movement with light resistance. Continue the back and forth motion of this recovery drill for 15-30 seconds.

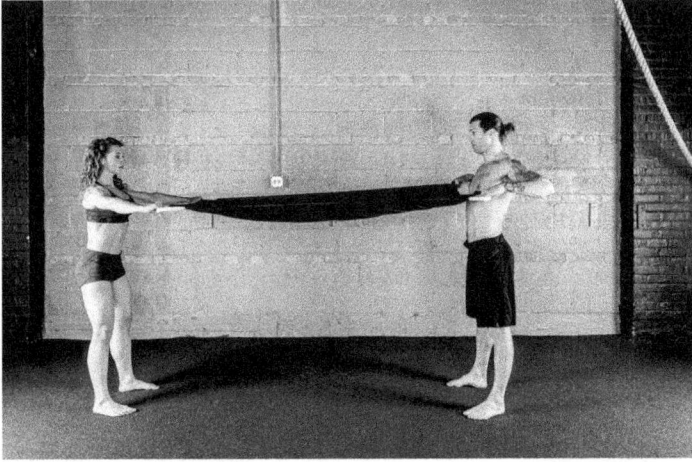

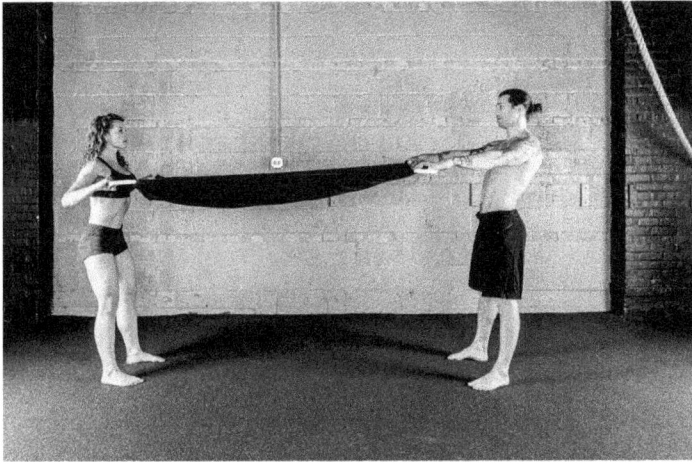

As you incorporate resistance recovery into your program, you'll see your conditioning and performance soar.

Surge Set Protocols

The following Surge Set protocols will give you a template to build your Commando Cardio workouts upon. Each protocol level has specific conditioning elements based on training ability. They include: exercise difficulty, rest intervals, number of Surge Sets per workout, and number of workouts per week. Eventually, you will want to create your own Surge Set protocols based on your conditioning levels and goals. I recommend starting at the beginner level and becoming proficient in each protocol before moving onto the higher levels.

Beginner Surge Set protocols

The beginner protocols should be performed 2-3 times a week.

Beginner level 1

Standing Overhand Velocity Swipe – 15-30 seconds

Rest Period – 60 seconds

Standing Underhand Velocity Swipe – 15-30 seconds

Rest Period – 60 seconds

Standing Overhand Velocity Swipe – 15-30 seconds

Rest Period – 60 seconds

Standing Underhand Velocity Swipe – 15-30 seconds

Beginner level 2

Standing Overhand Velocity Swipe – 15-30 seconds

Rest Period – 60 seconds

Lunging Overhand Velocity Swipe – 15-30 seconds

Rest Period – 60 seconds

Lunging Overhand Velocity Swipe – 15-30 seconds

Biceps Pull Resistance Recovery – 60 seconds

Standing Underhand Velocity Swipe – 15-30 seconds

Beginner level 3

Squatting Overhand Velocity Swipe – 15-30 seconds

Rest Period – 60 seconds

Squatting Underhand Swipe- 15-30 seconds

Rest Period – 60 seconds

Lunging Underhand Swipe – 15-30 seconds

Row Pull Resistance Recovery – 60 seconds

Lunging Underhand Swipe – 15-30 seconds

Biceps Pull Resistance Recovery – 60 seconds

Standing Overhand Velocity Swipe – 15-30 seconds

Beginner level 4

Standing Overhand Velocity Swipe – 15-30 seconds

Rest Period – 60 seconds

Kneeling Overhand Velocity Swipe – 15-30 seconds

Biceps Pull Resistance Recovery – 60 seconds

Kneeling Underhand Velocity Swipe – 15-30 seconds

Row Pull Resistance Recovery – 60 seconds

Scissor Jump Overhand Velocity Swipe Combo – 15-30 seconds

Biceps Pull Resistance Recovery – 60 seconds

Standing Underhand Velocity Swipe – 15-30 seconds

Beginner level 5

Squatting Overhand Velocity Swipe – 15-30 seconds

Biceps Pull Resistance Recovery – 60 seconds

Kneeling Underhand Velocity Swipe – 15-30 seconds

Row Pull Resistance Recovery – 60 seconds

Lunging Overhand Velocity Swipe – 15-30 seconds

Biceps Pull Resistance Recovery – 60 seconds

Lunging Overhand Velocity Swipe – 15-30 seconds

Triceps Extension Resistance Recovery – 60 seconds

Scissor Jump Underhand Velocity Swipe Combo – 15-30 seconds

Row Pull Resistance Recovery – 60 seconds

Scissor Jump Overhand Velocity Swipe Combo – 15-30 seconds

Intermediate Surge Set protocols

At the intermediate level, we increase the Surge Set to 30-45 seconds and will decrease the rest time to 30-45 seconds. The intermediate level protocols should be performed 3-4 times a week.

Intermediate level 1

Squatting Overhand Velocity Swipe – 30-45 seconds

Rest Period – 30-45 seconds

Jump Squat Overhand Velocity Swipe Combo – 30-45 seconds

Rest Period – 30-45 seconds

V-Straddle Underhand Velocity Swipe Combo – 30-45 seconds

Rest Period – 30-45 seconds

Scissor Jump Overhand Velocity Swipe Combo – 30-45 seconds

Rest Period – 30-45 seconds

Criss-Cross Jump Underhand Velocity Swipe Combo – 30-45 seconds

Rest Period – 30-45 seconds

Kneeling Overhand Velocity Swipe Combo – 30-45 seconds

Rest Period – 30-45 seconds

Lunging Underhand Velocity Swipe – 30-45 seconds

Rest Period – 30-45 seconds

Lunging Overhand Velocity Swipe – 30-45 seconds

Intermediate level 2

V-Straddle Overhand Velocity Swipe Combo – 30-45 seconds

Rest Period – 30-45 seconds

Criss Cross Jump Underhand Velocity Swipe Combo – 30-45 seconds

Rest Period – 30-45 seconds

Squatting Overhand Velocity Swipe – 30-45 seconds

Rest Period – 30-45 seconds

Jump Squat Underhand Velocity Swipe Combo – 30-45 seconds

Rest Period – 30-45 seconds

Kneeling Overhand Velocity Swipe – 30-45 seconds

Rest Period – 30-45 seconds

Criss Cross Jump Overhand Velocity Swipe Combo – 30-45 seconds

Rest Period – 30-45 seconds

Lateral Shuffle Underhand Velocity Swipe Combo – 30-45 seconds

Rest Period – 30-45 seconds

V-Straddle Overhand Velocity Swipe – 30-45 seconds

Intermediate level 3

Scissor Jump Overhand Velocity Swipe Combo – 30-45 seconds

Rest Period – 30-45 seconds

Scissor Jump Underhand Velocity Swipe Combo – 30-45 seconds

Rest Period – 30-45 seconds

Lunging Overhand Velocity Swipe – 30-45 seconds

Rest Period – 30-45 seconds

Lunging Underhand Velocity Swipe – 30-45 seconds

Rest Period – 30-45 seconds

Jump Squat Overhand Velocity Swipe Combo – 30-45 seconds

Rest Period – 30-45 seconds

Jump Squat Underhand Velocity Swipe Combo – 30-45 seconds

Biceps Pull Resistance Recovery – 30-45 seconds

Squatting Overhand Velocity Swipe – 30-45 Seconds

Row Pull Resistance Recovery – 30-45 seconds

Squatting Underhand Velocity Swipe – 30-45 seconds

Intermediate level 4

Criss Cross Jump Overhand Velocity Swipe Combo – 30-45 seconds

Rest Period – 30-45 seconds

Jump Squat Underhand Velocity Swipe Combo – 30-45 seconds

Rest Period – 30-45 seconds

Scissor Jump Overhand Velocity Swipe Combo – 30-45 seconds

Rest Period – 30-45 seconds

Kneeling Underhand Velocity Swipe – 30-45 seconds

Row Pull Resistance Recovery – 30-45 seconds

Lateral Shuffle Overhand Velocity Swipe Combo – 30-45 seconds

Biceps Pull Resistance Recovery – 30-45 seconds

Lateral Hop Underhand Velocity Swipe Combo – 30-45 Seconds

Row Pull Resistance Recovery – 30-45 seconds

Criss Cross Jump Overhand Velocity Swipe Combo – 30-45 seconds

Biceps Pull Resistance Recovery – 30-45 seconds

V-Straddle Underhand Velocity Swipe – 30-45 seconds

Intermediate level 5

Lateral Hop Overhand Velocity Swipe Combo – 30-45 seconds

Bicep Pull Resistance Recovery – 30-45 seconds

Lateral Hop Underhand Velocity Swipe Combo – 30-45 seconds

Triceps Extension Resistance Recovery – 30-45 seconds

Scissor Jump Overhand Velocity Swipe Combo – 30-45 seconds

Row Pull Resistance Recovery – 30-45 Seconds

Scissor Jump Underhand Velocity Swipe Combo – 30-45 seconds

Biceps Pull Resistance Recovery – 30-45 seconds

Criss Cross Jump Overhand Velocity Swipe Combo – 30-45 seconds

Triceps Extension Resistance Recovery – 30-45 seconds

Criss Cross Jump Underhand Velocity Swipe Combo – 30-45 seconds

Row Pull Resistance Recovery – 30-45 seconds

Jump Squat Overhand Velocity Swipe Combo – 30-45 seconds

Biceps Pull Resistance Recovery – 30-45 seconds

Jump Squat Underhand Velocity Swipe Combo – 30-45 seconds

Advanced Surge Set protocols

At the advanced level the Surge Set is increased to 45-60 seconds and the rest times are decreased to 15-30 seconds. Advanced Surge Set protocols can be performed 4-5 times a week.

Advanced level 1

Standing Overhand Velocity Swipe – 45-60 seconds

Rest Period – 15-30 seconds

Lunging Underhand Velocity Swipe – 45-60 seconds

Rest Period – 15-30 seconds

Lunging Overhand Swipe – 45-60 seconds

Rest Period – 15-30 seconds

V-Straddle Underhand Velocity Swipe – 45-60 seconds

Rest Period – 15-30 seconds

Scissor Jump Overhand Velocity Swipe Combo – 45-60 seconds

Rest Period – 15-30 seconds

Squatting Underhand Velocity Swipe – 45-60 seconds

Rest Period – 15-30 seconds

Squatting Overhand Velocity Swipe – 45-60 seconds

Rest Period – 15-30 seconds

Jump Squat Underhand Velocity Swipe Combo – 45-60 seconds

Rest Period – 15-30 seconds

Kneeling Overhand Velocity Swipe – 45-60 seconds

Rest Period – 15-30 seconds

V-Straddle Underhand Velocity Swipe – 45-60 seconds

Advanced level 2

Kneeling Overhand Velocity Swipe – 45-60 seconds

Rest Period – 15-30 seconds

Scissor Jump Underhand Velocity Swipe Combo – 45-60 seconds

Rest Period – 15-30 seconds

Squatting Overhand Velocity Swipe – 45-60 seconds

Biceps Pull Resistance Recovery – 15-30 seconds

Criss Cross Jump Underhand Velocity Swipe Combo – 45-60 seconds

Rest Period – 15-30 seconds

Kneeling Underhand Velocity Swipe – 45-60 seconds

Rest Period – 15-30 seconds

Lateral Shuffle Overhand Velocity Swipe Combo – 45-60 seconds

Row Pull Resistance Recovery – 15-30 seconds

Squatting Underhand Velocity Swipe – 45-60 seconds

Rest Period – 15-30 seconds

Lateral Hop Overhand Velocity Swipe Combo – 45-60 seconds

Rest Period – 15-30 seconds

Standing Underhand Velocity Swipe – 45-60 seconds

Criss Cross Jump Overhand Velocity Swipe Combo – 45-60 seconds

Advanced level 3

Scissor Jump Overhand Velocity Swipe Combo – 45-60 Seconds

Rest Period – 15-30 seconds

Criss Cross Jump Underhand Velocity Swipe Combo – 45-60 seconds

Biceps Pull Resistance Recovery – 15-30 seconds

Squatting Overhand Velocity Swipe – 45-60 seconds

Rest Period – 15-30 seconds

Jump Squat Underhand Velocity Swipe Combo – 45-60 seconds

Triceps Extension Resistance Recovery – 15-30 seconds

Lateral Shuffle Overhand Velocity Swipe Combo – 45-60 seconds

Rest Period – 15-30 seconds

V-Straddle Underhand Velocity Swipe – 45-60 seconds

Row Pull Resistance Recovery – 15-30 seconds

Lateral Hop Overhand Velocity Swipe Combo – 45-60 seconds

Rest Period – 15-30 seconds

Scissor Jump Underhand Velocity Swipe Combo – 45-60 seconds

Biceps Pull Resistance Recovery – 15-30 seconds

Criss Cross Jump Overhand Velocity Swipe Combo – 45-60 seconds

Rest Period – 15-30 seconds

Squatting Underhand Velocity Swipe – 45-60 seconds

Advanced level 4

Lateral Hop Overhand Velocity Swipe Combo – 45-60 seconds

Biceps Pull Resistance Recovery – 45-30 seconds

Lateral Shuffle Underhand Velocity Swipe Combo – 45-60 seconds

Triceps Extension Resistance Recovery – 15-30 seconds

Jump Squat Overhand Velocity Swipe Combo – 45-60 seconds

Row Pull Resistance Recovery – 15-30 seconds

Kneeling Underhand Velocity Swipe – 45-60 seconds

Biceps Pull Resistance Recovery – 15-30 seconds

Criss Cross Jump Overhand Velocity Swipe Combo – 45-60 seconds

Triceps Extension Resistance Recovery – 15-30 seconds

Scissor Jump Underhand Velocity Swipe Combo – 45-60 seconds

Row Pull Resistance Recovery – 15-30 seconds

Lateral Shuffle Overhand Velocity Swipe Combo – 45-60 seconds

Biceps Pull Resistance Recovery – 15-30 seconds

V-Straddle Underhand Velocity Swipe – 45-60 seconds

Triceps Extension Resistance Recovery – 15-30 seconds

Jump Squat Overhand Velocity Swipe Combo – 45-60 seconds

Row Pull Resistance Recovery – 45-60 seconds

Lateral Hop Underhand Velocity Swipe Combo – 45-60 seconds

Advanced Level 5

Scissor Jump Overhand Velocity Swipe Combo – 45-60 seconds

Biceps Pull Resistance Recovery – 15-30 seconds

Criss Cross Jump Underhand Velocity Swipe Combo – 45-60 seconds

Triceps Extension Resistance Recovery – 15-30 seconds

Jump Squat Overhand Velocity Swipe Combo – 45-60 seconds

Row Pull Resistance Recovery – 15-30 seconds

Lateral Shuffle Underhand Velocity Swipe Combo – 45-60 seconds

Biceps Pull Resistance Recovery – 15-30 seconds

Lateral Hop Overhand Velocity Swipe Combo – 45-60 seconds

Triceps Extension Resistance Recovery – 45-60 seconds

Jump Squat Underhand Velocity Swipe Combo – 45-60 seconds

Row Pull Resistance Recovery – 15-30 seconds

Lateral Hop Underhand Velocity Swipe Combo – 45-60 seconds

Biceps Pull Resistance Recovery – 15-30 seconds

Criss Cross Jump Overhand Velocity Swipe Combo – 45-60 seconds

Triceps Extension Resistance Recovery – 15-30 seconds

Scissor Jump Underhand Velocity Swipe Combo – 45-60 seconds

Row Pull Resistance Recovery – 15-30 seconds

Lateral Shuffle Overhand Velocity Swipe Combo – 45-60 seconds

Rest Period – 15-30 seconds

Front Split Underhand Velocity Swipe – 45-60 seconds

Rest Period – 15-30 seconds

Front Spit Overhand Velocity Swipe – 45-60 seconds

The "partner call" Surge Set

A fun and challenging way to perform Commando Cardio is the "partner call" Surge Set. Each partner will take turns calling out an exercise during the timed set. This will improve your reactive time and overall athletic ability.

Embrace the Pain and Reset your Conditioning Governor

"There are two primary choices in life: to accept conditions as they exist, or accept the responsibility for changing them."

-Denis Waitley

When I was younger, I used to enjoy going to a local entertainment spot that had batting cages, adventure golf, and go-carts. After a few cracks of the bat, it was time to race my friends around the go-cart track. I remember crushing the gas pedal to go as fast as possible. The problem is that the go-carts had a governor on the motor that controlled the speed. No matter how hard you press the pedal, the top speed was already set by the governor.

In the same way, our conditioning levels also have a governor. The governor in your body determines

You can reset your body's governor.

the limitations of your strength and conditioning based on what it thinks is safe. The good news is that you can reset your body's governor. The secret is to continually push the body past its perceived limits. As you progress through the Commando Cardio program, you will have to push yourself and get used to temporary discomfort. That is how transformation occurs.

Learning to embrace the pain leads to great gains. I have heard stories about people who are terrified of needles. Getting a vaccination or blood drawn is traumatizing for them. One of the techniques that is used to help these individuals overcome their fear was learning to embrace the temporary pain of the needle. They were taught to focus on welcoming the temporal pain of a vaccination in return for the healthy benefit of being immune to possible disease. The temporary discomfort was a small price to pay for good health. In the same way, the payoff from the temporal pain of continually reaching your lactic acid threshold during a Surge Set is incredible athletic conditioning levels.

Your goals will help you push through the pain. I remember the pain I experienced during several of the world record truck pulls that I performed with my mentor John Brookfield. The goal was to pull a 31,000 lb. plus semi-truck for the distance of one mile in as fast as a time possible. There were times when my lower back and quadriceps felt like they were on fire. The goal helped me push past the pain. I knew every step I took was one step closer to the goal. Temporary pain was the price I had to pay to get to the finish line.

What are your conditioning goals? Take some time to write them down before you

Specific goals lead to specific results.

start the Commando Cardio program. Just as a captain charts a ship's course toward its destination, you too should clearly write down where you want to go with this program. Too many trainees have general conditioning goals. General goals lead to general results. Specific goals lead to specific results. Statistics have shown that less than 3% of all people write down their goals. Maybe that's why so many people are frustrated when they aren't seeing the results they desire. Writing down your goals and reviewing them daily will give you the motivation you need to keep pushing your limits and resetting your governor.

START NOW!

"Don't wait. The time will never be just right."

-Napoleon Hill

A final reminder- don't wait until you have a Neuro-Burner to start the Commando Cardio program! You can start today! When I first read about kettlebells years ago, I wanted to train with them. I didn't have the money to purchase one. So, I went to the welder and had a plate loaded kettlebell handle made. Doing snatches with a plate loaded kettlebell was quite painful, but I wasn't going to let lack of equipment keep me from training. Eventually, through saving and some sacrifices, I was able to purchase my first 70 lb. kettlebell. It was a great investment; I still use it today!

I have always tried to get creative when it comes to equipment. When I wanted to start grip training, I couldn't afford thick barbells and dumbbells, so I bought a whole bunch of duct tape and wrapped it around the handles. I still have a pair of my home made thick (duct taped) dumbbells. I have lifted bricks, rocks, hardware store sandbags, blocks, and whatever else I could find to get stronger. The lack of equipment early on in my career inspired me to start my own strength equipment company.

In the early days of my strongman shows we didn't have much equipment either. I used to pack the bricks for breaking, steel bars, and everything else for the small-scale show in the back of our Dodge Caravan. I had no sound system, lights or all the other makings of a stage show. I used what I had, and now the show has grown so large it has to have a trailer to transport all the equipment.

The message is clear, do what you can with what you have. When you start to see the value of the Commando Cardio program, I am sure that you eventually will want to invest in a Neuro-Burner. You have the program to help you achieve amazing levels of conditioning. What are you waiting for?

The message is clear, do what you can with what you have.

You can get your Neuro-Burner and other great gear at www. neuropowersource.com.

Acknowledgements

To my Lord and Savior Jesus Christ

To my family

To John Brookfield and Ori Hofmekler for teaching me the importance of velocity training

To Rob Miller, Katie Peterson, and Mary Carol Fitzgerald for the outstanding photographs

To the entire team of individuals who worked on this project

About the Author

The exploits of Guinness World Record-holding strongman Jon Bruney have been immortalized in *Ripley's Believe it or Not, The Guinness Book of World Records*, as well as shown nationwide on NBC's *America's Got Talent, The Today Show*, ABC's *To Tell the Truth*, and TruTv's *Guinness World Records Unleashed*.

Thousands of people have personally experienced Jon's jaw-dropping Pressing the Limits motivational strength program. A true renaissance man in the realm of strength-development, Jon Bruney is a best-selling author, world-class trainer, coach, motivational speaker, strongman, and pastor. Jon's work with competitive athletes includes Olympians and NFL players.

He is the author of the best-seller *Neuro-Mass: The Ultimate System for Spectacular Strength* and *The Neuro-Grip Challenge: A Radical Program for Building Strength and Power in Your Upper Body*. He also wrote a training series called Foundations, featured in *MILO*, which was considered the world's most prestigious strength training journal.

Jon has been responsible for the design of numerous pieces of cutting-edge training equipment now in use around the world. Jon is a veteran of multiple trainer certification courses and was the first to achieve the grueling Battling Ropes Level II Certified status.

www.ingramcontent.com/pod-product-compliance
Lightning Source LLC
Chambersburg PA
CBHW051028030426
42336CB00015B/2778